Pastoral Care: Mental Health

Edna Hunneysett

All rights reserved, no part of this publication may be reproduced by any means, electronic, mechanical photocopying, documentary, film or in any other format without prior written permission of the publisher.

> Published by
> Chipmunkapublishing
> PO Box 6872
> Brentwood
> Essex CM13 1ZT
> United Kingdom

http://www.chipmunkapublishing.com

Copyright © Edna Hunneysett 2009

Chipmunkapublishing gratefully acknowledges the support of Arts Council England.

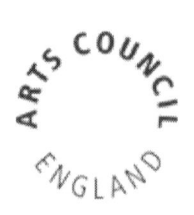

Acknowledgement

I acknowledge on completion of my study that I am indebted to many people.

I am grateful to various members of staff at the University of Durham, with special thanks to Professor Gyles Glover and Professor Stephen W Sykes for their time, patience, and help; to Doctor Dent of the University of Teesside; to the Royal College of Psychiatry; to the Vice Chair of the South Tees Local Ethics Committee; and to a Research Fellow of the North of England Institute for Christian Education, for advice given.

I thank all who participated in the pilot studies, all individuals of Christian congregations who responded to the questionnaire, and religious leaders and the Colleges who obligingly gave information on training programmes.

I thank Canon Eddie Gubbins for his interest and help, and Doctor Dan Donovan, for his support and encouragement.

Lastly, I acknowledge with deepest gratitude the support, patience and never-ending encouragement of my husband Ray, our children and grandchildren.

Edna Hunneysett

Preface

Jesus indeed cared... he fed the hungry, made the blind see, the deaf hear, the crippled walk... But by being surprised by all the remarkable things he did, we forget that Jesus did not... return the boy of Nain to his widowed mother without having felt her sorrow, that he did not raise Lazarus from the grave without tears and a sigh of distress that came straight from the heart. What we see, and like to see, is cure and change. But what we do not see and do not want to see is care, the participation in the pain, the solidarity in suffering, the sharing in the experience of brokenness.

In a community like ours we have put all the emphasis on cure. We want to be professionals: heal the sick, help the poor, teach the ignorant, organise the scattered. But the temptation is that we use our expertise to keep a safe distance from that which really matters... Let us therefore first ask ourselves what care really means and then see how care can become the basis of community.

When we honestly ask ourselves which persons in our lives mean the most to us, we often find that it is those who, instead of giving much advice, solutions or cures, have chosen rather to share our pain and touch our wounds with a gentle and tender hand. The friend who can be silent with us in a moment of despair or confusion, who can stay with us in an hour of grief and bereavement, who can tolerate not-knowing, not-curing, not-healing and face with us the reality of our powerlessness, that is the friend who cares.

Nouwen HJM (1974) *Out of Solitude: Three Meditations on the Christian Life*. Ave Maria Press, Indiana, 31–32, 34

Edna Hunneysett

Pastoral Care: Mental Health

Table of Contents

Acknowledgement

Preface

1 Introduction

2 Historical Development of Christian Theological Understanding of Insanity

3 A History of Developing Attitudes of Ordinary Christians Towards Insane People

4 Christian Activities in Contemporary Society Concerning People with Mental Illnesses

5 Contemporary Attitudes of the General Public Towards People with Mental Illnesses

6 A Survey of Pastoral Formation of Christian Leaders on Supporting People with Mental Illnesses and their Families

7 Methodology of Research of Attitudes in Christian Congregations

8 Comparison of Attitudes of Christians with Those of the General Public Towards People with Mental Illnesses

9 Research of Christian Attitudes Today Towards People with Mental Illnesses

10   Addressing Issues and Integration of People with
     Mental Illnesses in Christian Congregations

Bibliography

Chapter 1
Introduction

Behind this study lay a variety of personal experiences concerning people with mental illnesses, and their carers and families.

My mother experienced a serious mental illness, an obsessive-compulsive disorder, but it went undiagnosed for many years because, apart from myself in whom she eventually confided, she disclosed her secret to no one until latterly in her life. My early feelings of frustration and irritation changed over the years because of my gradual grasping of her condition. My attitude became one of acceptance and compassion, listening and care in proportion to the development of my understanding that what she was experiencing was a mental illness that caused her much suffering, tortuous at times. My conclusion in this instance was that understanding could help bring about positive reform in attitudes.

Our daughter was diagnosed with severe clinical depression at thirteen years of age due to a chemical/hormonal imbalance triggered off at puberty. She experienced relapses during her teen years. The intense devastation that mental illness brings upon an individual and which deeply affects those closest to them was highlighted for me while caring for our daughter throughout her teenage years. As her main carer, I personally experienced feelings of isolation, spiritual emptiness, and lack of pastoral understanding and support.

I have participated in a pastoral support group for people caring for those with mental illnesses for many years, and more recently have participated regularly in one for those experiencing mental illness. I have had numerous opportunities to listen to individuals, mostly in church settings, who have approached me after hearing me speak publicly, and have confided in me about issues surrounding mental health problems.

When employed full-time for eighteen months at a mental health day centre, (with more than eighty individuals on the register), I gained experience of how people with mental illnesses felt they were negatively viewed in the eyes of the world. For example, the introductory statement of "I am a nutter" conveyed one client's self-perception, and made me realise that it is this sort of labeling that stigmatizes and dehumanises a person.

My personal experience, of looking after our teenage daughter and supporting my mother, led me to think more deeply about pastoral care, and to question its availability to carers and families where there is mental illness. At the time, I was in the process of doing a degree in divinity, and I made a decision to continue studying in order to research this question. Consequently, as part of my Master's degree, I researched the nature of support available to carers especially of people with mental illness and Church involvement (Hunneysett, 1998).

The research for the Masters degree included examination of data collated from the responses to questionnaires by twenty-three carers of people with mental illnesses on their experiences and needs. It provided detailed information from four Roman Catholic clergy on pastoral care of sick people including those with mental illnesses, and their families and carers. On completion of this small study I still had unanswered questions.

My personal experience and knowledge accounted for a number of questions:
- Why had my mother felt unable to confide in anyone especially her general practitioner and her parish priest, her neighbors and friends, even most of her close family, about her illness?
- What lay behind the reason the priest gave for feeling unable to visit my sick daughter?
- Why did so many carers write or verbally communicate to me that they believed there was a need for more openness, more church support and understanding?
- Why was the client at the day center so readily able to introduce himself with a stigmatizing label?
- Why did the clients at the center feel "different?"

I had had expectations that, if ever we had a child who was seriously ill, the Church would be there for us. I had witnessed evidence of this with other families, with other illnesses.
- So was it the fact that it was a mental illness that my daughter was experiencing that made the difference?
- Was there a lack of confidence, in spite of wanting to help, by clergy and laity?

This led to further questions:
- Bearing in mind the concept that a person with a mental health disorder can be experiencing an illness is a fairly recent one, are people with mental illnesses seen as needing pastoral care like other sick people?

- Is the message of Christianity to be compassionate, to love and care for one's neighbor as oneself, delivered by Christian congregation leaders, inclusive of people with mental illnesses and their carers?
- Is it taken for granted that Christians will know what kind of support people with mental illnesses and their families might need?
- Are Christian leaders informed and trained in this area of pastoral care?
- Do denominations differ in their training of leaders?
- Do Christian denominations focus on different perspectives concerning mental illnesses?
- Are attitudes of the general public, Christian or otherwise, the same towards people with mental illnesses, or does being a Christian make a difference?
- Are there differences between Christian denominations on attitudes and understanding towards people with mental illnesses?
- If research demonstrates that there is need for improvement in attitudes and pastoral care, how is this to be achieved?

With these questions in mind, I decided to embark on further research to see if I could come to some answers, although I am aware that there are more questions here than can be adequately tested in a study of this size.

This current research is a completely new piece of work, not comparable with my previous research work but a progression of it, and a genuinely new work on attitudes in Christian congregations investigated statistically.

Pastoral Care: Mental Health

The subject matter concerns contemporary attitudes in Christian congregations towards people with mental illnesses. My initial approach was to draw up and issue questionnaires to members of the three denominations with the aim of statistically comparing their attitudes with those of the general public; of comparing the attitudes of different Christian denominations; and of investigating beliefs into possible causes of mental illnesses with reference to religion, and whether Christians considered themselves more prone to mental illness because of their religious beliefs. There was a section in the questionnaire on suggested methods of addressing issues concerning mental illness in order to increase awareness and understanding, and of ways that might possibly improve the integration of people with mental illnesses into Christian communities.

As background to this empirical work, I surveyed the history of the Christian Church's theological understanding of insanity from secondary sources in order to highlight those influences on attitudes that may have implications for today. I also surveyed the history of the attitudes of ordinary Christians so as to place contemporary Christian attitudes in context. I report my investigation of Christian involvement today and, through a literature search, contemporary attitudes in society. After these preliminary chapters, I report the results of a survey on pastoral formation of church leaders. I explain the methodology of my research, and follow this by presenting the main part of the empirical work. This includes discussion and application of the research including material from case studies. Recommendations conclude the study.

Key terms are used in this work without definition: for example, "insanity," "madness," "illness," *et cetera*, and no distinction is made. The words are used interchangeably and not in a technical sense.

The next chapter presents the findings of my survey into the historical development of the Christian Church's theological understanding of insanity. What does my investigation reveal?

Chapter 2
Historical development of Christian theological understanding of insanity

Madness has always been and remains an elusive thing, but Porter (1987) tells us that, while all societies make arrangements for dealing with people who display weird behavior, the people demonstrating the peculiarities are dealt with quite differently from society to society and from era to era.

Before the nineteenth century, according to Porter (1997), treatment of mad people hardly constituted a specialist branch of medicine. Neugebauer (1978) cites psychiatry appearing as a medical speciality only at the end of the eighteenth century. Jones, however, places it even later as a twentieth century specialism and adds, that before the middle of the eighteenth century, "the frame of reference for the study of insanity does not exist" (Jones, 1993: 13). Shorter (1997) agrees that before the end of the eighteenth century there was no such thing as psychiatry, but mental disorder as such had always been familiar; psychiatric illness is as old as the human race; and the human society has always had ways of coping with it. The process of Christian theological developments concerning insanity and mental disorders must therefore be placed within the context of the time and not from a contemporary perspective.

Supernatural intervention

Theologians of the early Christian era attributed bizarre actions to divine intervention (Graham, 1967).

In the ancient world there was widespread belief in spiritual powers or beings that existed in addition to well-known gods and goddesses. These beings were not understood as being necessarily evil, though some might have been. There are traces of the belief in harmful spirits in the Old Testament writings, but the belief that there existed numerous evil spirits or demons and with a leader, evolved in the late postexilic period. The idea expanded that there were armies of demons, under the leadership of Satan or the devil, doing battle with God and God's allies. Eventually the notion developed that demons could invade human bodies and personalities and cause madness, physical disease, or other specific problems. Such ideology as this "is clearly reflected in the synoptic Gospels of the New Testament, where Jesus is known as one who characteristically exorcises demons (e.g. Mt. 8:28-34; Mk. 5:1-20)" (Achtemeier, 1985).

There were two main traditions of how the Greeks made sense of madness. One described it as sickness of the soul (as expressed by the arts); alternatively, explanations were given, drawn on physical causes and effects. Evidence for the first is found in the inner conflicts of guilt feelings and grief presented in the tragedies; and the classification of mania and melancholy as disease is an instance of the second tradition. The culture of Medieval Latin Christendom absorbed and made use of both of the Greek alternatives, "madness as moral trauma, and madness as disease" but fitted them within a "cosmic Christian scheme, madness as divine Providence, which could impart a higher significance to either" (Porter, 1987: 12-13).

Evidence that in early Christianity it was thought that evil spirits could cause disease is demonstrated by a number of stories of demon possession in the New Testament (Avalos, 1999). However, Toner (2004) is of the opinion that, even if some disease generally accompanied demoniac possession, Christ and the Evangelists did not necessarily equate possession as the cause. He gives the event in Luke 13:32 as an example where Christ distinguishes between the expulsion of evil spirits and the curing of disease.

According to Graham, Origen (c.185-254), a convert to Christianity, a biblical scholar and an influential writer, held that sickness, injury and mental disorders were "correlated positively with demons" (Graham, 1967: 21). Jackson (1972) insists that there was such a "diagnosis" as possession. In one form or another this ubiquitous notion, he says, had been known to antiquity as an explanation for disease and other misfortunes, and certain welcome experiences. Then, in later antiquity and the early Middle Ages, it was taken up by the Christian Church and adapted to Christian ideas of good or bad supernatural influences.

The idea of good and bad supernatural influences for strange behaviour gave rise to the problem, when people were manifesting religious delusions, of whether they were under the influence of God or possessed by the devil. If the condition of possession was considered to be genuine, those who were thought blessed were honoured. There are numerous accounts of mental states in medieval literature that were considered to be distinctly unusual, but those affected did not see themselves as ill or mentally disordered and were not usually considered as such by others. Some were considered ascetics, and others, prophets, holy men, or mystics (Jackson, 1972). According to Graham (1967), Christian theology was able to treat madness in quite distinctive ways; for example, in seeing mental disorder a sign of war for the possession of the soul waged by God and Satan. Medieval and Renaissance minds expanded this in being able to regard madness as religious, moral, medical, divine, diabolical, good, or bad.

Pattison (1989) states that there has been great diversity of ways of looking at and treating mental disorder down the centuries, and relates to this the importance of the religious and supernatural significance attached to the disorders through much of human history. Graham (1967) concludes that Judaism and Christianity both accepted that evil spirits were a reality and consequently tried to suppress occultism, as they believed that humankind had been endowed with a free will, and perverse behaviour was seen as a voluntary submission to the forces of the devil.

Not every theologian thought in this way in medieval times. For example, Abelard (1079-1142) ridiculed the idea that the devil caused insanity, but his way of expressing his opinions "was so bitter that the Catholic Church denounced him" (Graham, 1967: 61). Duns Scotus (c.1265-1308), a member of the Franciscan Order, on the other hand, was an example of those who were emphatic that mental disorders were linked with Satan.

Exorcism

The possibility of possession by evil spirits required a response by the early Christian Church.

Evidence from medical theology of Mesopotamian cultures suggests the idea was pervasive that illness was caused by supernatural beings and that it affected both king and commoners. Exorcism was a means used to address this. There are letters between "Esarhaddon and his exorcist" about the king's anxiety and in one letter, an "exorcist" tries to comfort Esarhaddon. Two principal strategies, sometimes overlapping, were used to deal with the medical theology that some unknown being was the instigator or controller of the illness. One was to pray to all possible gods or beings possibly responsible for the illness in the hope that the right one would be located so as to plead with it. The other was to entreat a divine intermediary to locate the being responsible for the malady and following this, a proper ritual could be carried out (Avalos, 1995).

According to Toner (2004), the Egyptians ascribed certain diseases to demons and resorted to magical incantations as a means of expelling them. Babylonian magic was tied up with medicine, and as some diseases were attributed to a kind of demonic possession, exorcism was considered the easiest way of curing them. A god or goddess would be invoked to call out the evil spirit and repair any damage that the being had caused.

The Israelite health care system had its own history. In the Ugaritic Kirta Epic there is a king, Kirta, who is not well. According to Avalos (1995), his illness is depicted as a kind of demon that must be "beaten and expelled." The being appointed goes to the king's house and expels the malady. There is no example in the Old Testament of evil spirits being expelled by a human being. For example, it is an angel in the Book of Tobit (Tb. 8:3) who took the devil. In extra-canonical Jewish writings there are recordings of demons being exorcised by incantations (Toner, 2004).

According to McNeill (1953), exorcism for insanity, epilepsy, and other diseases was widely practiced in the early Church. The most common mode of therapy practiced for addressing possession was exorcism; that is the driving out of the spirit in a non-physical manner (Lerner, 1997). Rahner and Vorgrimler (1983) explain that underlying the natural chain of events in nature and history, there is a supernatural dynamism of diabolically evil powers that does not eliminate natural causes but employs them for its own objectives. They see no real dilemma between overcoming the phenomenon by exorcism, a solemn prayer to God in the name of and sanctioned by Christ and the Church for protection against evil powers, and by medicine. This primary meaning of exorcism in Christian usage is a "strictly religious act or rite," but in ethnic religions, exorcism as a religious act is more often replaced by magical or superstitious means, as the use of protective means against evil spirits has always been a part of these religions (Toner, 2004).

No superstitious means were used in the very early Christian centuries; only a solemn prayer addressed to the evil spirit in the name of Christ. Sometimes other symbolic actions were used, for example, the laying on of hands or making the sign of the cross, as the latter was the easiest way of expressing faith in Christ crucified or invoking his divine power. At an early Christian time, the practice was introduced whereby candidates for baptism were exorcised, not with the understanding that they were possessed, but because of original sin, were prone to the power of the evil one from whose dominion they were to be delivered, a "symbolic anticipation of one of the chief effects of the sacrament of regeneration" (Toner, 2004). The Church still practices most of these ancient rituals for baptism.

Suicide

There were other theological concerns that had bearing on insanity in early Christianity. One in question was that of the salvation of people who committed suicide.

From very early Christian times, the Church firmly repudiated suicide. This was recalled recently when, in the United States Court of Appeals for the Ninth Circuit, findings were given relating to the rejection of physician-assisted suicide as a constitutional right (*Amici*

Curiae, 2004). In the report, it is written that suicide within the early Christian Church was not morally accepted. The report cites a number of early Church leaders, for example, Clement of Alexander (ca.155-220), Tertullian (ca.160-220), Basil of Caesarea (ca.330-379), Jerome (ca.342-419), Chrysostom (349-407), and Ambrose (ca.339-397), who condemned the practice of suicide (Larson and Amundsen, 1998). The report adds that as Christianity spread throughout the Roman world, the public rapidly became intolerant of the practice of suicide.

Augustine of Hippo (354-430) gave his theological reasons for the condemnation of suicide, and his influence in western theology has been immense. Augustine discusses whether suicide is an acceptable action. He argues that there is no injunction or permission in scripture to commit suicide for reasons of either ensuring immortality or of avoiding or escaping any evil. He denies self-destruction because of the commandment: *Thou shall not kill*. Augustine concludes that a valid reason for suicide does not exist and he reiterates, "that suicide is a detestable crime and a damnable sin, as the Truth plainly declares" (Bettinson, 1972: 32-39). Augustine's reasoning on victims of suicide and salvation was later manifest at the Council of Braga (563) when suicide was condemned as a crime, and any individuals who took their own lives were consequently denied a Christian burial. No matter under what conditions suicides took place or whatever the status of the person committing the act, individuals who committed suicide were buried away from their community. Added to this, their bodies were pierced with a stake "to offer protection against their malevolent souls" (Lipsedge, 1996: 40).

Over a century later at the Council of Toledo (693), the penalty of excommunication was imposed on any persons who attempted to do away with their lives, and suicide was denied as a means towards martyrdom. Suicide was a civil and religious crime in Tudor and Stuart England. Not only was the person, who had committed suicide, denied a funeral and burial in the churchyard, but also the dead person was tried posthumously and his movable goods were forfeited to the king's almoner. According to MacDonald (1981), it was only in the eighteenth century that the act of suicide came to be regarded as sufficient evidence of insanity. Graham (1967) concedes that Augustine held noteworthy ideas about suicide but, in such cases, feels he confused these with the role of mental disorders.

There were developments in understanding mental disorder in the twelfth century that helped initiate changes with relevance to suicide and mental derangement. An extension to Church law decreed that a person could be punished only if he willingly committed any illegal act and, therefore, a deranged person who tried to commit suicide was exempt from excommunication (Graham, 1969). On the other hand, Aquinas (c.1225-1274) echoed the Church's severe attitude with reference to suicide by referring to it as the most fatal of sins, his reason being that it could not be repented of. In his *Summa Theologiae*, Aquinas (1969) propounds that suicide is wrong for three reasons; in the first place it runs counter to the inclinations of nature and charity to oneself; it does injury to society to which each human person belongs as part of a whole; and finally, it wrongs God who gives the gift of life and who alone has the authority to take it.

In the Middle Ages, it was standard clerical teaching that suicide took place because of temptations of the devil (Lipsedge, 1996). In the late sixteenth and early seventeenth centuries, "traditional religious beliefs reinforced the view that people who committed suicide were fully rational beings" (MacDonald, 1981: 133-134). Clergymen and most of the laity upheld the medieval insistence that suicidal behavior signaled as alienation from God. The determination to kill oneself was seen as giving in to temptation and giving up hope of salvation, despairing of God's mercy.

Human rationality

Another theological concern that had bearing on insanity in early Christianity was the definition of what was meant by being human.

Aquinas' definition of humanity in relation to the faculty of reason was a possible influence. According to Aquinas, human beings are set apart from other animals because they have minds and are in God's image in virtue of their intelligent nature. That is to say, it is only in a rational creature that there is a resemblance to God and "what puts the rational creature in a higher class than others is precisely intellect of mind." Human beings achieve a likeness to God in their understanding (Aquinas, 1964: 90-102).

Inquisition, witchcraft and demonic possession

In the Middle Ages, there was another event that had bearing on the treatment of insane individuals. In 1232, the Church set up the Inquisition, the juridical prosecution of heresy by special ecclesiastical courts (Livingstone, 1990).

The traditional meaning of heresy, rigorously defined in medieval canon law, is the formal denial of any defined doctrine of the faith (Richardson and Bowden, 1983). Pope Gregory IX (c.1148-1241) had entrusted the Inquisition to the Dominican Order, and largely from the Dominican and Franciscan Orders, appointed papal inquisitors. Innocent IV (d.1254), reigning Pope from 1243, allowed the use of torture by the Inquisition (Livingstone, 1990). The persecution of heretics by the inquisitors became entwined with another phenomenon that was emerging, that of witchcraft, described as the exercise by individuals of supposedly being in communication with Satan or evil spirits. The different unusual phenomena described as witchcraft had resemblances to what could be described as mental derangement.

The writings in the First Book of Samuel (1S. 28:7, 25) and the condemnation of witchcraft in the Book of Exodus (Ex. 22:18) in the Old Testament, and the Letter to the Galatians (Ga. 5:20) in the New Testament, have been suggested as proofs of the existence of witchcraft. The persecution of witches had been part of Roman law but was discouraged in the early Middle Ages. However, popular superstition had not died out. Dealings with the devil were considered heretical. Towards the end of the thirteenth century, at Toulouse, the earliest execution of a witch took place because she had supposedly confessed to certain relations with the devil. Within two centuries, these kinds of witchcraft fantasies reached the most unimaginable proportions, and great numbers of individuals were accused of witchcraft. Two Popes allowed the inquisitors to deal with those accused of witchcraft, if connected with heresy, and secular courts also took action.

Shortly after the invention of printing (in the mid-fifteenth century), the *Malleus Maleficarum* document, translated as the *Hammer of Witches*, written by two Dominicans, Kramer and Sprenger, was published, and it became the tool of the Inquisition. Graham gives his understanding of the events. This publication received the endorsement of Pope Innocent and King Maximilian and with these approvals, Kramer and Sprenger proceeded to the Faculty of Theology at the University of Cologne and persuaded the reluctant professors to give their approval. The Letter of Approbation includes the following.

> *In the year 1487… the power of making search and inquiry into all heresies, and especially the heresy of witches… granting them every faculty of judging, and proceeding against such even with the power of putting malefactors to death….* (Graham, 1967: 78).

Porter (1997) affirms that the late medieval church warned against the Devil and evil spirits, that women were considered particularly susceptible to Satan, and that during the next three hundred years thousands were executed. According to Koenig (2005), historians disagree on the extent to which insane persons were persecuted during this time although, he adds, there is no doubt that such persecution occurred, resulting in many deaths.

Tritheim, a Benedictine Abbot of Sponheim in West Germany from 1483-1506 was, according to Graham (1967), very humane in his attitudes apart from his witchcraft fantasies. Tritheim felt that there should be more inquisitors to deal with the witches whom he believed had very bad diseases; that people died as a result of their evil; and that they were not aware that they were bewitched. Although mass persecutions began in the late fifteenth century, the Reformers with often "exaggerated belief in the power of the devil, further contributed to the evil" (Livingstone, 1990: 558). It was in 1684 that the last witch was hanged in England (Hunter and MacAlpine, 1963).

Koenig reports that "the widespread belief in Europe that demons or evil spirits were the cause of symptoms in some people with mental illness" was brought to the New England colonies (Koenig, 2005: 117). He states that belief in demonic possession had become so strong in Europe, and later in the American colonies that violent action was taken to rid the population of such persons with many burnt at the stake as witches or sorcerers. The last witch-hunts in the United States took place in Massachusetts in 1692, and these included executions.

Influential people and writings

There were other more clinical developments in progression from early Christian times as well as a record of some guidance and instruction that was influential in addressing insanity.

Towards the end of the fifth century, for example, about fifty years after Augustine's death and after the fall of Rome, the onset of a new empire produced "several figures who approached clinical problems with some degree of sophistication" (Graham, 1967: 31). One of these was Aurelianus (c.420) from Rome and Carthage, a man of compassion and kindness to patients with mental distress, and who disapproved strongly against using chains to restrain them (Jackson, 1972). Among other medical writers of importance was Paul of Aegina (625-690), a Greek doctor living in Rome, who recommended gentle treatments, including music, for those with mental derangement, but there was some allusion to satanic possession (Porter, 1997).

In Medieval Europe, Bacon (c.1214-1292), a Franciscan friar, made an outstanding contribution to the evolution of human thought that was of immense value to individual mental health. He argued that the disorders were not supernatural, was against the idea of demonic possession, and held that much ascribed to demons was from natural causes (Graham, 1967).

Another major influential writer was Aquinas (1975) who wrote on the degrees and level of incapacity of mental disorders. The motivation for this was the necessity of distinguishing between the various categories of feebleminded and unstable persons whom the Church was accustomed to baptize. He focused on Canon Law and, in determining the categories, included those who had at one time been sane but had suffered the loss of reason.

The teaching of an English Franciscan Friar, Bartholomew Angelicus, Professor of Theology in Paris, in the thirteenth century, was influential, especially from a Christian perspective, in developing understanding of insane people. He compiled a manual, first printed in 1470, and translated into English in 1495, that was designed to help priests and their parishioners in their ministry to insane people (Hunter and MacAlpine, 1963). Graham holds that Bartholomew's influence remained alive long after he had died and his manual was translated into five modern languages before the invention of printing, and the manual was also used in schools of theology. It continued to be used for several hundred years.

Another example was Vives (1490-1540), born in Valencia and author of *De Subventione Pauperum*, who believed that hospitalization, and humane treatment, was the way to help those classed as insane. Paracelsus, (1493-1541), a Swiss physician, was also amongst those who opposed the popular theory of demons as the cause of illnesses (Graham, 1967).

There are records that show evidence of continued interest in this area in a further number of writings. For example, in 1550, Pope John XXI (d.1277) had a text *Folk Remedies against madness*, published. Some identical text had appeared in another sixteenth century book, first published in 1539 by Moulton, a Dominican Friar, that had been reprinted fourteen times by the 1560s.

Boorde (1490-1549) a Carthusian monk and suffragan bishop of Chichester as well as a physician, had his first book published in 1547 and his second in 1552. He separated as demoniacs, a group of violent or suicidal victims who might need exorcism, over and above the standard remedies for madness. Hunter and MacAlpine (1963) add that, interestingly, he devoted the section on treatment to domestic management because, in his day, Bethlem Hospital was the only institution for insane persons in the country and this with accommodation for only about twenty patients.

Another example was of some clinical developments shown in the writings of Weyer, physician and Rhinish reformer. In 1563, Weyer had published an expose of the folly of witchcraft rejecting the popular belief in demons without equivocation. Weyer agreed that people who had lost their power of reason would be open to any crime and, consequently, that it was horrendously erroneous to torture witches. He advocated treating those considered to be witches with compassion and empathy; and that those sentencing them to the burning at the stake were butchers.

Oldhams, a Jesuit satirist of this era, likewise agreed that the idea of witches was a myth. However, Bodin, a Catholic publicist and economist, who had had published *De la Demondomanie des Sorciers* to prove the existence of sorcerers, vehemently disagreed with

Weyer's enlightened view, and responded by adding a long chapter to his own publication in order, albeit unsuccessfully, to try and prevent witch-hunting of the sixteenth century from disappearing into obscurity (Graham, 1967).

A further example of opposition and clinical development is found in the work of Scott (c.1538-1599), who was repeatedly confronted with cases of supposed witchcraft. His careful observation of these sorts of people convinced him that they were not demonically possessed but insane, and had published *The Discoverie of Witchcraft* (1584), in which he strengthens his argument by stating that witchcraft was contrary to reason, scripture and nature. This enlightened humanitarianism was a major advance because Scott identified a large section of insane people who were eventually rescued from theological conjecture and statutory prosecution and brought within the domain of natural sciences (Hunter and MacAlpine, 1963).

However, James I, on his accession to the English throne, had his book *Daemonolgie in Forme of a Dialogue*, already published in 1597, republished in London in 1603 in order to reaffirm witchcraft so as to counteract the enlightened views of Scott. Following this, a witchcraft Act of 1604 replaced a milder one, which meant that many of the severities were revived. Long term, however, it prefaced progress as it eventually instigated change. The objective study of mental disorder was beginning, although it was slow progress for those who challenged the attitudes of the public, the legal system and the Church authorities (Graham, 1967).

Some Christian writers continued to influence progress. These included Bright (c.1551-1615), a physician to St. Bartholomew's, London (1585-1591) and subsequently an Anglican priest, who wrote *A Treatise of Melancholie* (1586); Downame (d.1652), a puritan divine of London and preacher of God's word, who published in 1600; Wright (1561-1623), a Jesuit priest, who published in 1601; Reynolds (1599-1676), King's Chaplain and Bishop of Norwich, published in 1620; and Baddeley (1586-1670) in 1622 (Hunter and MacAlpine, 1963).

During the late sixteenth and the seventeenth centuries, melancholy became fashionable and this in turn nurtured the belief that suicidal behavior, rather than being seen as a religious crime, was instead viewed as a mental disorder (MacDonald, 1981). The same view is to be found in Sym (c.1581-1637), a country clergyman, who wrote a treatise, *Life's Preservative against Self-Killing* (1637), in which he also advocated that not all individuals who committed suicide were sinners to be damned, but that many were sick in mind and not responsible for their actions.

Taylor (1613-1667), Bishop of Down and Connor, wrote *The Rule of Conscience* (1660) concerning scruples. The writings, published in 1691, of Rogers (1658-1728), a nonconformist minister, were particularly valuable, "because they were written from personal experience" (Hunter and MacAlpine, 1963: 248). Another example is that of Moore, chaplain to William and Mary, bishop successively of Norwich and Ely, who had a sermon *Religious Melancholy* published in 1692, and this book went into seven editions, which showed, according to Hunter and MacAlpine, that it filled a real need.

Exorcism continued to be a contentious issue especially after the division of Christianity after the Reformation. MacDonald (1981) explains that in the late sixteenth century, Protestant reformers, because of exorcism being linked to Catholic liturgies, objected to its use and eliminated it from the Church of England's liturgy. Dissenting sects continued to exorcise people in their belief that Satan possessed such people. The Jesuits, during the reign of Elizabeth, exploited the church's reluctance about the use of exorcism by "touting their own traditional power of exorcism as proof of their superior spiritual authority" (MacDonald, 1981: 206). The Anglican hierarchy apparently did little to counter this until the Puritan wing of the church developed a method of casting out devils by group prayer and fasting, but this was forbidden by a canon enacted in 1604.

Eventually, from the second half of the seventeenth century, Church leaders had become very disheartened by the carnage and chaos caused by the unceasing conflicts over good and evil spirits (Porter, 1987). Increasingly, the manifestations of witchcraft came to be interpreted, at least by the social elite, essentially as misconceptions, the results of individual and shared hysteria, the work of uneducated, self-deluding minds. The persecution practically came to an end in the eighteenth century under the influence of the Enlightenment.

The Enlightenment and further writings

The European Enlightenment of the eighteenth century marks a watershed in the developing understanding of madness and mental disorders. This had repercussions on the Christian theological understanding in this field.

The fundamental notions of The Enlightenment included a commitment to reason as the proper tool and final authority for determining issues, a stress on nature and the appeal to what is "natural," and a rejection of the authority of tradition (Richardson and Bowden, 1983). It was an intellectual revolution that deeply affected Christianity, as it is crucially linked to fundamental Christian values in the progress of a society towards a greater freedom, tolerance and maturity (Rahner and Vorgrimler, 1983).

Porter (1997) describes therapeutic developments that included the theory and treatment of insanity undergoing a "seachange." For example, the notion of insanity as demonic possession was finally discredited among medical men, and in the courts. It was argued that disorders such as mania and melancholy were not caused by supernatural intervention but that insanity was organic. Porter believes that there was now benevolent sympathy towards insane people but only through first seeing them as very different from the rest of society. He depicts a similar process of redefinition afoot within Christianity itself.

Suggested evidence of this changing understanding was in the example of the Spital Sermon, preached in 1718 by Snape (1675-1742), chaplain to Queen Anne and George I, in Saint Bridget's church in Easter week. According to Hunter and MacAlpine (1963), this deserves a special mention because it was the first in which "Distraction" was discussed from a medical point of view as well as theologically. Koenig (2005) affirms the rapid increase of nonreligious explanations for mental disorders.

The repeal of the Witchcraft Acts in 1736 had officially ended the waning belief in demonical possession as far as the civil power was concerned but, as stated by Hunter and MacAlpine (1963), there was still a trace of the uncanny and fearsome in connection with mental disorders, the lingering notion that it was possibly the devil at work or punishment for sin.

MacDonald (1981) agrees that, while throughout the eighteenth century the governing classes were repudiating supernatural explanations of causes of insanity, ordinary people continued to believe in witchcraft and demonology.

In order to help counteract this, Farmer (1714-1787), a theologian and minister of religion, published *An Essay on the Demoniacs of the New Testament* (1775) to try to help people understand that those referred to as "demoniacs," in the Scriptures, were people with mental disorder or epilepsy (Hunter and MacAlpine). Similarly, with regard to understanding of suicide, Moore (1743-1811), rector of Cuxton and vicar of Boughton-on-Blean in Kent, penned a most extensive treatise *A Full Enquiry into the Subject of Suicide* (1790) on the "natural, social, moral and religious" aspects of suicide. A secularized view of suicide in favor of medical explanations was developing. Again, Pargeter (1760-1810), physician and specialist in insanity and subsequently a naval chaplain, in his publication *Observations on Maniacal Disorders* (1792), was the first, according to Hunter and MacAlpine, to detail an account of how much could be achieved by both by both "management" and the influence of the physician. These latter writings, from the early eighteenth century, were published around and after The Enlightenment period, and its influence is evident in the writings. By the late eighteenth century, causes of suicide were deemed by physicians to be entirely physical or psychological (Lipsedge, 1996).

Psychiatry and religion

Over the course of the nineteenth century, practitioners became known as psychiatrists, and the profession as it is known today came into being.

In the early nineteenth century, patients were increasingly integrated into the asylum "community," and as the century progressed, numbers soared of patients detained in institutions. According to Lerner (1997), the comfortable familial home had given way to a series of enormous, bleak institutions that often contained as many as several thousand patients in dreadful conditions.

Growing attention was given to the outward appearances of mentally ill patients, such that many late nineteenth psychiatrists came to believe that hysteria and other mental and nervous ailments were recognizable by particular external signs or "stigmata." Also, in the late nineteenth century, hypnotism was to some extent a new dynamic psychiatry that appeared on the scene (Kleinman, 1980). Lerner explains that it was linked to the scientific exploration of mediums and spiritualism allowing for the aspects of the psyche to be investigated by physicians.

Freud (1856-1939) developed new concepts, the outcome of which was psychoanalysis treatment (Cole, 1997). He was one of many psychiatrists who developed psychogenic theories in the early twentieth century, thus abandoning the hypnoses previously used (Lerner, 1997). Koenig (1997) states that Freud was considered the father of modern psychiatry, who argued convincingly that religion was linked to neurosis, and his negative attitudes towards traditional religious beliefs and practices had widespread effects on the mental health field. According to Koenig, Ellis, founder of the Rational Emotive Therapy Institute in New York later in the twentieth century, identified eleven characteristics of religiosity that Ellis believed ran counter to sound mental health. Koenig adds that Watters, in Canada, emphasized that Christian doctrine and teachings were incompatible "with the primary components of sound mental health." Thus it appeared, Koenig states, that many prominent mental health professionals of the twentieth century believed that religion had either no influence or a negative one. By the end of the twentieth century, "the negative attitude towards religion expressed by Freud and other contemporary mental health professionals such as Waters and Ellis had impacted the personal views of many practicing psychologists and psychiatrists" (Koenig, 2005: 27). Koenig adds that psychiatrists in England were even less likely than those in the United States to have religious beliefs.

Pastoral education and training

In the twentieth century, there were more developments in theology relevant to mental disorders.

For example, in America in 1925, Dr. Anton Boisen began a relatively new venture both in psychiatry as well as in theological education (Bruder, 1953). An educational program was the means by which disciplined training, initiated by the Reverend Boisen, Father of the Clinical Pastoral Education movement, linked trainee clergy and mental health. He placed theological students in supervised contact with people in mental institutions. Boisen himself struggled with mental illness but his religious faith had enabled him to use his experiences "to make lasting contributions to the care of those with similar problems" (Koenig, 2005: 80). In the 1930s, the integration of religion and psychology for psychotherapeutic purposes began, forming the American Foundation of Religion and Psychiatry. The role of pastoral counseling evolved over the years from spiritual counseling to pastoral psychotherapy, thus integrating theology with the behavioral sciences (American Association of Pastoral Counselors, 2004).

Clinical theology was an influential development in the mid twentieth century especially in pastoral training of clergy. It included in its forte mental disorders. Lake was a doctor, psychiatrist and an active Evangelical Christian whose mission was to heal the individual in body, mind and spirit. This led him to search for a fusion of the disciplines of psychology and theology that eventually became known as Clinical Theology (Christian, 1991). Christian, who had been associated with the Clinical Theology Association for more than twenty years, edited a publication drawing on Lake's many lectures, articles, sermons, newsletters (to the members of the Clinical Theology Association), and seminars and conferences led by him.

Lake's original intention was to set up an in-service pastoral training system for the clergy. In 1959, the Scottish Pastoral Association (SPA) was formed to strive to bring together ministers, doctors and social workers. The first issue of its journal *Contact* appeared in 1960. Around this time, some Universities were introducing diplomas in pastoral studies. Lake was the founder of the Clinical Theology Association instigated in 1962, and in the same year a Clinical Theology Center was established in Nottingham where he gathered a team round him. Together, part of their work was training clergy in an increasing number of seminars around the country. The network of people and organizations in the development of pastoral care and counseling became the Association for Pastoral Care and Counseling. In 1966, Lake's *Clinical Theology* was published, the contents of which, reflected the mind of a man who made his "own uniquely significant contribution to pastoral care and education in Britain" (Christian, 1991: xi). Clinical theology was important in its time, but it failed to exert a wider influence on pastoral care in its subsequent demise.

Other influences in the mid twentieth century were encyclicals that emerged from the Second Vatican Ecumenical Council (1962-1965) as these included teaching relevant to pastoral ministry to people with mental illnesses. Broadly speaking, any persons undergoing any form of suffering need temporal support and spiritual nourishment alongside their families.

The teaching, for example, makes clear that the Church recognizes Christ in those who are suffering and strives to do all it can to relieve their need (Flannery, 1987: LG8). Another example is of the Church expressing its solidarity with the whole human family, that each individual should be considered as a whole person in body, soul and mind, and that a human person is a social being who can only live and develop in relationship with others. Everyone is therefore called to look upon their neighbors as themselves, to respect every person, to enable all to live in a dignified way, and to come to their aid in a positive way (Flannery, 1987: GS1, 12, 31-32). A further document reinforces Christian values on how to treat people with illness and suffering. In it, the Church decrees that wherever people are racked by misfortune or illness, Christians in charity should comfort them with devoted care and assist in whatever way is necessary to relieve their needs (Flannery, 1987: AA8).

In 1972, the Church issued further instructions on developments in pastoral care of sick people. Anyone involved in helping sick people should to do whatever is deemed necessary to help them both physically and spiritually (Flannery, 1982: HD4). This fulfills Christ's command, as it was Christ's intention that concern is aimed at helping the whole person and to offer both physical relief and spiritual comfort, and the Church admonishes an imitation of the kind of concern that Christ himself showed.

John Paul II enunciated further teachings in 1981. The Christian family is called to give witness of "generous and disinterested dedication to social matters, through a 'preferential option' for the poor and disadvantaged." Love goes beyond those of the same faith and knows how to discover the face of Christ in each individual, especially in those who experience poverty, or who are weak and those who are suffering. Priests and deacons are admonished to support the family in its difficulties and sufferings and a prudent pastoral commitment, modeled on Our Lord, is called for in those families who find themselves in difficult situations (Flannery, 1982: FC47, 64, 73, 77).

In 1981, further instructions urged Christians to stand alongside organizations to foster support and increase initiatives to help alleviate suffering. Individuals, handicapped in any way, and their families, belong to the whole human family but may be in a minority. This may entail insufficient interest and added to that is "the often spontaneous reaction of a community that rejects and psychologically represses that which does not fit into its habits." People do not want to face negative aspects of life but this gives rise to exclusion and discrimination and, therefore, this tendency must be countered by education. The Church gives a reminder that the quality of a society and a civilization is gauged by the respect shown to the weakest of its members. Furthermore, it teaches that it is necessary to reflect on the distressing situation of the many people who undergo stress and shock that disturb their psychic and interior life, and it is important that the health of the spirit is fostered so that a person is not damaged in his deeper needs. Those responsible for planning programs in social care and integration of disabled people should make the family the starting point, as families need to be given great understanding and sympathy so as to help prevent feelings of isolation and rejection. The witness that these families give to the dignity, sacredness and value of the human person deserve open recognition and support by the whole community. Also, professionals and volunteers who give themselves to the service of the disabled should "learn to dialogue with the parents and families" (Flannery, 1982, The International Year of Disabled Persons, 1:3, 11:3, 5-6, 15, 13:11).

This teaching was brought together in a further publication in 1994 where specific reference is made to human misery being depicted in various ways, including to psychological illness. "The duty of making oneself a neighbor to others and actively serving them becomes even more urgent when it involves the disadvantaged, in whatever area this may be" (John Paul II, 1994, CCC 2448, 1932).

Ahead of the World Mental Health Day, 2001, the Pope, when speaking of those who are mentally ill, advocated that society must defend their rights and dignity. He reiterated that the Church looks with respect and affection on those who suffer such illness, and he exhorted everyone to welcome them, and to give special attention to those who are the most poor and abandoned (John Paul II, 2001). Pope Benedict XVI, in his message, *Mental Illness: A Real and Authentic Social Health Care Emergency* (Vatican City, 2005) given in Adelaide, Australia in 2006 (for the fourteenth World Day of the Sick), calls the attention of public opinion to the problems connected with mental disturbance, that afflict one-fifth of humankind, and exhorts Church communities to the commitment of bearing witness to the tender mercy of God towards those who are mentally ill.

This concludes the survey of historical development of Christian theological understanding of insanity, ending in the twentieth century with a more holistic approach in pastoral care, of mind, body and spirit, being advocated.

I continue, by presenting in the next chapter, a survey of the history of developing attitudes of Christian laity and ordained persons towards insane people. How did those at grass roots level, down the centuries, address this area of need?

Chapter 3

A history of developing attitudes of ordinary Christians towards insane people

Throughout antiquity, insanity provoked divergent responses that paved the way for lasting controversy. This is no less true for Christians.

Whether the stricken individuals were presenting frightening behavior verbally or in actions, languishing in despair, thought possessed by the devil, or being made destitute and resorting to begging, these individuals needed a Christian response and this would have posed a very difficult problem for Christians. Down the centuries, according to Koenig (2005), people of faith, (whether acknowledged or not), have sought to free those suffering mental disorders, or at least walk with them on their difficult journeys.

Christian charity

Throughout the history of Christianity, there is shown to be not only practical compassion towards those who were deranged, but also prayer for them. There is evidence of concern and support by clergymen.

In early Christianity, the public did not make itself responsible for the custody of a mad individual, but instead, the family had to look after the person in question and make sure that no one was harmed (Clay, 1909). Insanity was a family responsibility with the seriously disturbed individual being restrained at home, while others were allowed to wander. However, these individuals were feared and avoided because it was thought that the evil spirits within them might leave and enter another person (Porter, 1997). Thus, some of the insane people in medieval England were just left to their own devices and these deranged beggars were a common part of the medieval landscape as they wandered from place to place, community to community, in search of alms (Scull, 1993). Persons who suffered from symptoms of mental disorder were usually dealt with, firstly, and often only, by close members of their families, with physicians ministering to just a minority. Folk beliefs, superstition-ridden notions, religious, and other supernatural explanations were all used in an attempt to understand their conditions (Jackson, 1972).

So the picture throughout the Middle Ages, and later, is that it was rare for any special formal provision to be made for people who were considered to be insane, except within the family, or under the watch of the village community, or just being allowed to wander. Yet, Porter (1987) believes, that this old intermingling of mad persons with people at large possibly preserved some sort of common humanity. He sees it as being linked to Christian teachings in that it could have helped to maintain some sense of the mad person as a fellow human being, made in God's image, the same as all other believers. According to Porter, it would be inappropriate to deplore the indifference as especially cruel or to praise it as especially enlightened because it was simply that the traditional state was very limited in undertaking any welfare functions. In a larger community, there may have been an increased possibility of orthodox medical care; in a rural community, folk medicinal care was more common. Where the Church had influence, the Christian tendency to charity and care for one's neighbors would have overridden class and cultural differences (Jackson, 1972).

Pastoral Care: Mental Health

Christians resorted to prayer and intercession as specific ways of responding to the problem of mentally deranged individuals. For example, with regard to some mental disorders, Christians sought cures from God through direct prayers or through the intercession of saints and for healing by use of their relics. This happened in the cases where natural and supernatural causes other than possession were considered to be responsible for the maladies. Jackson (1972) believes that folk healers would have probably treated some, with the emphasis on medicines and with the frequent addition of magical practices or Christian prayers. During the early part of this period, faith healing would have been part of the Church's response.

An example of a seventh century saint as an intercessor associated particularly with mental health is Dympna, who fled from Ireland to Gheel in Belgium to escape from her father. He followed her, had the pastor who was protecting her murdered, and because Dympna insisted on resisting his advances, her father had her beheaded. According to the legend, several insane people who observed these terrible events were "shocked into sanity." Following from this event grew a family-care plan (Graham, 1967). A hospice built in Gheel to house insane people proved to be too small and many of them lodged in village households. Porter (1997) describes this as being like a family colony where the villagers looked after these people. Similar models of family care were started in Germany and France. In 1939, in the USA, a shrine to St. Dympna was built in Massillon, Ohio (Koenig, 2005). Dympna's life has been documented, and centuries later she is still prayed to as an intercessor, demonstrated in *The Litany of St. Dympna*, "Special patron of demented persons, pray for us" (Verne, 1961: 203).

Shrines were places of pilgrimages for insane people. According to Clay, some persons considered to be possessed were taken to holy places in the hope that the evil spirits might be expelled. There is an early thirteenth century window at Canterbury that shows an insane person who has been taken by his friends to the health-giving shrine of St. Thomas and is pictured tied with ropes, and being beaten with birch-rods. In the second scene, "he appears in his right mind, returning thanks, all instruments of discipline cast away" (Clay, 1909: 31). Even as late as the sixteenth century, Clay ascribes to reports of pilgrimages by insane people, especially to holy wells.

A person with the mental disorder or those close to him were more likely to turn to a priest or some other religious person for help (Jackson, 1972). The parish clergy had, for centuries, helped those with psychological disorders, and preachers used to instruct the people to "interpret emotional turmoil in religious and moral terms" (MacDonald, 1981: 176). Before and after the Reformation, the clergy would act as mediators between people with mental disorders and the rest of the community, and they provided the consolation and advice that the afflicted people needed greatly when they had acute anxiety attacks.

Monasteries and institutions

Very early in the Church's history, monasteries provided a place of refuge for sick people. This study uncovered a variety of institutions that have been recorded as providing shelter down the centuries for insane people, and of the Christian Church being involved in setting up places of asylum long before the eighteenth century. This was during the time when the word "asylum" was the term given to place of refuge from the unsympathetic world outside (Jones, 1993).

In the monasteries, medicine was included in the general education activities. It was because of promulgation by Benedict of Nursia (c.480-550) that infirmaries became part of the monastery establishment so that those monks who were ill could be cared for with kindness. Consequently, "monasteries served as seedbeds for the development of the Christian emphasis in the virtue of caring for the sick," and monks and brothers played an important role in the care of sick people (Jackson, 1972: 265). Also, certain monasteries and religious houses in Catholic countries traditionally cared for insane people (Kleinman, 1980; Porter, 1997).

There is record of the existence of a hospital in very early Christian times that made provision for deranged people. Basil the Great (c.330-379) was responsible for the erection of a town hospital that included in it a special place for insane people, demonstrating, according to Graham (1967), that Basil and a small group of Christians were definitely sympathetic towards mentally deranged individuals. However, no further details are given. Other reports refer to these kinds of institutions that were for the care of the infirm and destitute and were England's inheritance for over a thousand years. Hospitals were ecclesiastical, not medical institutions, and as such, were more inclined to care rather than cure. There were upwards of seven hundred and fifty such charitable institutions in Medieval England, and the earliest of these were houses of hospitality. There are, according to tradition, at least two hospitals or hospices that were founded in the tenth century, and two other early houses of charity are attributed to the Saxon bishops Oswald, and Wulstan of Worcester (c.1009-1050). In these, all sorts and conditions of persons were lodged, wayfarers, invalids, and even lepers, and during the twelfth century, more independent foundations became common (Clay, 1909).

It is possible to deduce from Clay's description of "ecclesiastical institutions" harboring "the destitute" and "wayfarers" that deranged beggars would have been given refuge. As early as the thirteenth century, insane people were being accepted as sick people and treated in general hospitals (Graham, 1967).

An example of an institution for the care of the infirm and the destitute is St. Bartholomew's hospital. The hospital and priory of St. Bartholomew were established simultaneously. According to Clay (1909), all needy people, the insane invalids together with those with weak or diseased bodies, were admitted into hospitals such as St. Bartholomew's of Smithfield. Around the year 1148, it was known as the resort of sick pilgrims including victims of insanity. The early inmates often came from considerable distances and, in the twelfth century, mad people were constantly being admitted to St. Bartholomew's. Wilmer and Scammon (1954) report from the Book of the Foundation of St. Bartholomew's Church in London, published at the eighteenth hundredth anniversary of its founding. In it, facts pertaining to the hospital make reference to cases of mental disorders and to the spiritual ethos.

An example of an institution abroad was of one in Spain, built on the outskirts of Valencia, and notable for its care of insane people. Dominguez (1967) records some details of this institution. Jofre (1350-1417), a priest in the Mercedarian Order (also known as the Order of Our Lady of Ransom), was inspired to found it in 1409. Seeing urchins mistreating a madman had motivated Jofre to preach a sermon about the encounter, and from this, citizens, aware of his message, were moved with compassion and initiated support to have a hospital built for the care of insane people. This resulted in the Hospital of Innocents, and in 1410, Benedict XIII issued a Papal Bull encouraging to people to support the new hospital financially. At this hospital, according to Dominguez, the patients were viewed as ordinary human beings experiencing a natural disorder. They were not seen as being possessed by the devil, nor was demonic possession understood to be the cause of any mental derangement. The kind treatment they received was their best therapy. The example shown by this Institution was followed in many cities in Spain, and with more of these hospitals being founded in Mexico and Rome.

Koenig (2005) reports that John Cuidad (1495-1550), born in Portugal to devout religious parents, as an adult experienced "an acute psychological breakdown." In the mid 1500s, he was the instigator of a hospital that emerged in Granada. It became one of the first facilities for those with mental health disorders in that part of the world. Cuidad was known as John of God, and after his death a movement of compassion spread across Spain to help poor, sick, and mentally disordered people. Two Orders emerged from his workers, and today, the work continues across forty-eight countries, worldwide.

A number of authors have written on a particularly renowned hospital in England that housed insane people. The priory of St. Mary of Bethlehem was built in 1247, firstly as a general hospital, but it began to admit insane people in 1403, and eventually became known as Old Bedlam. Most madhouses in London like Bethlem, before the close of the eighteenth century, had their origin as religious or municipal charities (Kleinman, 1980). Those patients who recovered were allowed to return to the community who were then responsible for them.

There are plenty of authors who vouch for the cruelty that was deemed to take place at Bethlem. For example, Lerner (1997) describes it as being dubbed "Bedlam" in popular parlance, a place synonymous with chaos, suffering and mismanagement. Bedlam, according to Graham (1967), eventually became the byword for cruelty and included a viewing gallery where patients were exhibited to entertain the public. While this inhuman practice of treating these people took place in England, it was also common in other countries, especially in Vienna. The admission in 1753, Koenig (2005) states, was two pence. This was such a lucrative venture for the hospital that the practice of displaying mad people did not end until the latter half of the eighteenth century. The conditions found at Bethlem, from an investigation in the early nineteenth century, according to Scull (1993), were appalling, that the patients were treated like "animals."

However, not all literature espouses this point of view, at least with reference to Bethlem Hospital. According to Allderidge (Bynum *et al,* 1985), precious little is known about Bedlam and much of what is known is a myth. Allderidge believes that whatever is thought about the treatment that took place at the hospital, for most of its history, the hospital was "largely geared to the concept of curability." There are references to cures by the blessings of God that suggest evidence of prayer, and the notion that Bethlem cured people was well known outside its walls. There is record of a request to the Bridewell chaplain to say prayers with the inmates, Bridewell and Bethlem being jointly administered from 1557.

Scull (1993) confirms that, until the seventeenth century, Bethlem was the only specialized institution of this kind, and what was offered in it was on an exceedingly modest scale. The reason for this is that in health care provision in England, the sixteenth century brought a major setback. The dissolution of the monasteries and chantries resulted in the closure of almost all the medieval hospitals that had offered at least shelter to those who were old, to sick people, and to those who were incapacitated. A few of these institutions survived the Reformation and were re-established on a new secular basis. St. Bartholomew's and St. Thomas's passed to the City of London after the Dissolution, as did Bethlem for treating mad people (Porter, 1997).

The Reformation
The Reformation had a major practical impact on the provision of resources for the poor people including those who were insane.

After the religious persecutions and changes of the Reformation period in Western Christendom between the fourteenth and seventeenth centuries, the development of witchcraft delusion and the decadence of hospitals, resulted in the serious neglect of insane people. Graham (1967) cites Catholic countries as being much less affected by the witchcraft delusion than the reformed countries, and that this was evident in the care that they showed towards deranged people. For example, hospitals in Italy and Spain went on to provide better care for them than hospitals in those countries that had been unsettled by the religious conflicts.

However, the dissolution of the monasteries, chantries, religious guilds and fraternities in the 1530s and 1540s had radically reduced the existing sources of charity. The real aid that they had provided for those in poverty was, according to Slack (1988), more considerable than has often been supposed. Discrimination between different categories of impoverished people had a tradition that stretched back to the thirteenth century and, by 1500, the dividing line between those whose poverty was considered to be acceptable as opposed to being undeserving had already been defined. The perception was that poverty stricken individuals were outside rather than inside society. They were on the margins of the community.

Neugebauer (1978) has a different point of view. He insists that his research indicates quite clearly, that in many areas of daily life, individuals with psychiatric disorders were viewed as physically ill and received kind and considerate attention. Evidence showed that cases dealt with were across a surprisingly broad spectrum of the social class and not just those of the privileged elite. On the other hand, Scull (1993) argues that it was precisely the rich mad people who came under the rule of the Courts of Wards and Liveries. Another aspect Neugebauer believes is that, in the histories of insanity, macabre scenes of witch-hunts and witch burnings have commanded great fascination, but that the existence and activities of an institution like the Court of Wards have been neglected.

Prior to the County Asylums Act in 1828 in a society preoccupied with the problems of sheer survival, most individuals undergoing a mental disorder were simply passed unnoticed (Jones, 1993). Insane victims had, according to Oxley (1974), been a burden on the poor rates from the earliest days and, as one of the categories of poor people, had always been a difficult group. Interest in insanity quickened about 1580, although the contemporary ideas were rooted in ancient science and medieval Christianity, and management of mental disorders did not change fundamentally before 1660. The social importance of the family was recognized in the arrangements for looking after mad and troubled people with financial relief for families as a way of helping the impoverished insane members. Private institutions did not begin to proliferate until the last half of the seventeenth century, and municipal asylums to rival Bedlam were not founded for another century.

The class of poor people continued to be dealt with on a local, parish level but were acknowledged to be more of a secular rather than a religious responsibility under the Poor Law Act of 1601, and people with mental disorders were simply one group among many who received the support. According to Scull (1993), one of the origins of the madhouse system, as far as pauper lunatic people were concerned, was the practice that developed from the mid-seventeenth century onwards of boarding them out, at the expense of the parish, in private dwelling houses. These abodes gradually became known as "mad" houses, but among the more affluent classes, the relatives of insane persons were frequently placed in the charge of medical men or clergymen.

However, Porter (1987) believes that before the eighteenth century, only a small proportion of people judged to be mad were confined in madhouses as they were mostly taken care of by their family or by a charity or by their parish. There was no attempt made to separate insane people from other vagrants and beggars in most workhouses or poorhouses. It was by an Act of Parliament in 1714 that these impoverished mad people were separately named and distinguished from disorderly persons. A further Vagrancy Act in 1744 added the clause that they should be cured, although how this was to be done was not specified. However, this was the origin by the public authorities of a commitment to treatment (Jones, 1993).

During the course of the seventeenth century, according to MacDonald (1981), religious contention and the shock of revolution hastened the triumph of medical explanations for insanity among the ruling classes, and in eighteenth century England, insanity was seen as a medical and social problem. On the other hand, Oxley (1974) believes that the plight of insane people was not understood and, as a result, they aroused fear and hatred rather than compassion and sympathy which is the reason he gives why so many who were accommodated in workhouses being chained up or placed in cells. If turned out of their homes, mentally deranged victims joined the many beggars who wandered the roads of early modern Europe. This is why it was the family and not the community who had to look after them with the result that, in England at least, such peoples if not shackled in their own homes, might be fastened to a stake in a workhouse or poorhouse (Shorter, 1997), workhouses having been established because of the Acts of 1722 and 1782 (Oxley, 1974). Jones (1993) gives a variety of means by which mentally deranged persons in the eighteenth century were accommodated. She lists workhouses and poorhouses, prisons, private madhouses, a few subscription hospitals, their own homes, or failing these, they wandered as vagrants.

It was not until the second half of the eighteenth century that the first attempts were made, according to Oxley (1974), to establish public institutions in the provinces where mentally deranged persons might be cared for in accordance with their "peculiar requirements." Institutions founded during the eighteenth century while more and more concentrating on sick people, also catered for persons deranged, orphans, and old people.

For example, Guy's hospital had established a ward for incurable lunatic people in 1728. St. Luke's hospital was established in London in 1751 and subsequently, other charity asylums began operating. They were not very large but their primary importance was the fact that they helped to legitimate the idea of institutionalization "as a response to the problem posed by the presence of mentally disturbed individuals in the community" (Scull, 1993: 18-19). However, according to Porter (1987), the biggest growth sector for the confinement of mad people before the nineteenth century was the private madhouse, and not until 1774 were any legal safeguards put in place to protect the inmates contained in these places.

It was primarily after the eighteenth century that mad houses became medical centers. Oxley (1974) argues that the voluntary lunatic asylums had shown that something could be done for insane people, that there was much more needed to be done, but that for many, nothing would be done until the relief authorities could be compelled to send their local mad people to asylums and pay for them. The County Asylum Act of 1808 legislated this. Jones (1993) argues that, after witchcraft and sorcery had died out, and most people had lost faith in exorcism, the only means of help for those with mental disorders that had any credibility was the support of the medical practitioners with their traditional methods, until the development of moral management.

There was an accelerated lessening of the Church's role in civil society and, a consequence to this, a change in attitudes towards dependence in society at large, "with a growing sense of the unworthiness of some of the recipients of aid" (Scull, 1993: 12). The benevolence of parish authorities replaced the charity of neighbors as neighborly charity, and it became formalized and compulsory by means of various inequitable handouts, and social control of the movements and settlement of those in need (Slack, 1988).

It was in the eighteenth century that mental disorder and the treatment of it came under the umbrella of an essentially physical viewpoint and, according to Pattison (1989), there was almost complete withdrawal of religious interest in and concern about mental disorders. Since that time, the Christian interest and contribution in this field of human experience, he believes, has been limited to intermittent spates of enthusiasm.

Although the rise of psychological medicine has often been represented as a saga of scientific progress, Macdonald (1981) argues that it was not. He believes that it was, instead, a story of religious hatred, political conflict, social antagonism, and finally, intellectual advancement. As for insane people, the eighteenth century, he feels, was a disaster, as they were confined to madhouses, to asylums, or even workhouses and prisons, and there was a wait of over a hundred years before there was any significant improvement by the medical profession in the methods of curing mental disorders.

New ideas in the late eighteenth century about people with mental disorders retaining their ability to reason, were surfacing. This was, according to Lerner, the realization that they were human beings who could and should be helped, in marked contrast to the preceding period in which, Lerner believes, "the madman's alleged lack or reason, reason being the crucial faculty which accounted for human uniqueness, served to justify treatment of him as inferior" (Lerner, 1997: 148).

Moral management and reform

From the late eighteenth century in particular there was a spread of all types of special dwellings for insane people, and these included "retreats managed by monks and nuns within Catholic Europe" (Bynum *et al*, 1988: 2). Alongside these, individual campaigners advocated reform.

One such Christian institution was The Retreat at York. In the late eighteenth century, The Retreat was founded in England where a different approach was initiated concerning treatment of people with mental health disorders. A number of authors contribute to documentation covering this institution, set up in 1792 because the local Quaker community decided to establish its own charitable asylum. Christians played a more manifestly significant part in this because The Retreat's founder was a Quaker layman, Tuke, who initially employed staff of his own faith. It was at this institution that growth of a movement known as "moral management" was instigated, and it developed independently in Britain through the example of The York Retreat. The work of Tuke was seen as opening a new chapter in the history of treatment of insane people because of the declared aim to give them the dignity and status of sick human beings (Hunter and MacAlpine, 1963).

Tuke was determined that those with mental health disorders at The Retreat would be treated with humanity and without physical restraint. Jepson, a well known Quaker and faith healer, was appointed as head attendant. Tuke and Jepson's model of care included acknowledging that every patient was essentially human (Nolan and Crawford, 1997). Pattison (1989) acknowledges that Tuke's fundamental philosophy was that, if you recognize the God-given humanity within these people and treat them accordingly, they are more likely to recover. Tuke also declared, according to Scull (1993), that in opposition to what was surmised, madmen had not completely lost their reason; it was distorted rather than obliterated. Digby (1985) believes the firm conviction held by those who ran The Retreat, that insane people did not lose their essential humanity, enabled these Friends to be responsive to the feelings of patients and their friends and relatives. The importance of spiritual values was emphasized, and the everyday care of the patients was seen as a combination of medicine and religion. Jones describes The Retreat as being unique because it developed a form of treatment based, not on the meager medical knowledge of the time, but on "gentle Christianity and common sense" (Jones, 1993: 26).

According to Scull (1993), statistics collected during The Retreat's first fifteen years suggested that moral treatment could bring about the healing of a large proportion of insane individuals from their disorders. A central fact about moral treatment was that it highlighted that the most obnoxious features of existing mad houses were really unnecessary cruelties. Even more so, it helped towards bringing about the end of these abuses (Lerner, 1997; MacDonald, 1981). William Tuke's grandson, Samuel Tuke (1784-1857), publicized The Retreat's success story in 1813. Hunter and MacAlpine (1963) believe that this book by a layman did more to improve the care and treatment of insane people in asylums than many of the writings by physicians.

However, respectable mad doctors did not, according to MacDonald (1981), introduce the moral therapy movement into common practice until the end of the eighteenth century. Attempts to construct institutions such as The Retreat only began in the second half of the eighteenth century, as did that of asylums like those at Manchester and Liverpool (Oxley, 1974). This moral management of therapy was an important new development exercised in the asylums of the nineteenth century (Pattison, 1989).

Early American psychiatry was heavily influenced by this development in England. The Quakers took the moral therapy movement to America in the early 1800s and it soon became the dominant form of psychiatric care with Institutions springing up in Philadelphia, Boston, New York and Connecticut (Koenig, 2005). Similarly in France, from 1838, each department had to erect an asylum for the impoverished insane people.

There is record of other individuals in this country and abroad, apart from Tuke, who advocated for reform, but abuses remained despite regular inspections (Kleinman, 1980). Crusaders emerged to try and expose these and campaign for better conditions. In France, for example, Pinel (1745-1826), a progressive reformer and physician as well as a devout Roman Catholic, took responsibility for insane people at Bicetre in 1793 (Kleinman, 1980; Porter, 1997; Hunter and MacAlpine, 1963). According to Kleinman, Pinel believed insane individuals behaved like animals because they were treated as such, and he is credited with liberating insane people from the restraining treatment and transferring them from confinement to care (Cule, 1997). This message was favorably received by all those who strove for social and humanitarian reforms of which there were many in the early nineteenth century England (Hunter and MacAlpine, 1963). McNeill states that the reforms introduced by such as Pinel in France, Tuke in England, and Benjamin Rush in America, began a slow work of transformation, and those individuals, mentally afflicted, were "once more regarded as fellow human beings" (McNeill, 1953: 60).

In Europe, the post-Renaissance era produced other Christian-minded individuals who left their mark on mental health. For example, Rabelais, priest, doctor and teacher, had an enlightened humanistic approach and steadfastly opposed the abuse of those deemed to be insane (Graham, 1967). Another example was Chiarug (1759-1820) working in Florence, who advocated replacing cruelty with kindness (Kleinman, 1980; Porter, 1997). Dorothy Dix campaigned in America for better conditions for mentally ill people and was also influential in Europe, including England and Scotland (Koenig, 2005).

In the 1820s, there was a great reform in the Swedish mental hospital system. The first Swedish psychiatrist came from a family of which most members were active in the Moravian evangelical movement and, because of the influence of evangelism amongst several of the reformers, insane people were no longer condemned. They were understood to be unhappy or neglected individuals whose lives could be improved with Christian love and fatherly education (Qvarsell, 1985).

Another example was Conolly (1794-1866), an outstanding early Victorian British psychiatrist who, while stressing moral therapy, also agreed with the physical basis of insanity (Kleinman, 1980). He was noted for his introduction of non-restraint, and had published *Treatment of the Insane without Mechanical restraints* in 1856. According to Jones (1993), he provided a very good example of how the asylum doctors were developing their skills.

The Seventh Earl of Shaftesbury (1801-1885), a fervent Evangelical and for many years the president of the British and Foreign Bible Society, was another campaigner who worked with tireless energy to make sure that adequate asylum facilities were established (Jones, 1993). This great humanitarian reformer was so impressed by the model of care at The Retreat, that he endeavored, unsuccessfully, to establish a network of asylums throughout England.

Secularization of institutions

It was after 1808 that county lunatic hospitals were established (MacDonald, 1981; Porter, 1997; Kleinman, 1980). Some Christian activity concerning people with mental disorders was evident in the twentieth century.

Porter (1987) questions whether mentally disturbed individuals confined to a madhouse in 1650, 1750, or 1850, received treatment any worse than others still wandering abroad or shackled in a barn. He feels it would be a mistake to depict the movement to institutionalize mad people as essentially repressive as he feels it was principally segregation. In time, experience increasingly proved, according to Porter, that insane persons did not recover as had been predicted, and the asylum, far from being the instrument of regeneration, became a place where those thought to be incurable were detained. The great majority seen by mad doctors or psychiatrists in the two centuries after 1750 had been excommunicated from their fellow humans and set apart in special institutions with their legal rights and personality removed. Society has progressively defined itself as rational and normal, and by doing so, had sanctioned the stigmatizing and exclusion of those alienated or excluded from society. McNeill states that the "secularization of the institutions for insane people apparently drove out of them most elements of compassion and humaneness" (McNeill, 1953: 59), that in the eighteenth and early nineteenth centuries, it was common practice to chain insane inmates permanently to the floor.

During the nineteenth century, the institutionalization of people with mental derangement became increasingly the concern of the state. The original purpose of the asylums, according to Barham (1992), were "reformatories," but as the pressures of Victorian society increased, the asylums provided a refuge for people who did not have a social place in society. They became "custodial" rather than "curative" institutions, with psychiatric ideologies providing a convenient shield to deflect searching moral questions about the social fate of vulnerable groups of people. In the second half of the nineteenth century, the whole endeavor went out of control, and the asylums became massive, overcrowded, stigmatized institutions (Jones, 1993). By 1900, the optimism for curability, with which the nineteenth century had opened, had almost entirely evaporated. In time, the asylum became a repository, a kind of receptacle warehouse, for those deemed unfit to participate in normal society (Kleinman, 1980).

There was evidence of Christian concern in the early twentieth century, in the founding of the Guild of Health (1904) to promote the Church's Ministry of Healing. Its objects included bringing together Christian people, including doctors, psychologists, and ministers of religion, to work in fellowship for fuller health, both for the individual and the community. This was to enable all members to study the interaction between physical, mental, and spiritual factors in well-being; and to sustaining and strengthening by prayer, sick people, those who minister to them, and all who exercise the divine gift of healing (Holmes, 2002).

By World War I, asylums, according to Shorter, had become huge receptacles for very mentally disturbed people, but he points out, that for the increase in numbers, families would first have had to decide to send them away. Originally, Shorter argues, distracted relatives of poor families were kept at home or turned out and some did inflict afflicted relatives onto the Church. However, in upper-class families they were most commonly kept at home, and yet, in the nineteenth century, there was willingness for the wealthy to send their relatives away. Shorter believes it was a change in families that contributed to this, with "a new style of family life," for which mental derangement in a beloved member was "no longer possible to behold" (Shorter, 1997: 51). Another point he makes is that what was biological psychiatry for doctors, was a question of nerves for patients. Patients found the notion of suffering from a physical disorder of the nerves much less disturbing than knowing that their disorder was insanity. Porter (1997) believes that The Great War was a watershed, endorsing the realisation in society that health was a national concern; this confirmed by a Ministry of Health being established in 1919.

After the end of the First World War, conditions were beginning to improve again, and asylums were increasingly being called "mental hospitals." Outstanding among these was the Maudsley Hospital, completed in 1915. In 1918, the Board of Control drafted a report for the Government. It included a recommendation that the Board should be empowered to make grants for after- care work by voluntary societies, a reference to the Mental After-Care Association formed in 1879. The chaplain of the Middlesex asylum published two articles in the *Journal of Mental Science* on the subject, and stressed the need for some form of follow-up care for discharged patients. The outcome of the Royal Commission of 1924-26 included the point that that "it has become increasingly evident that there is no clear line of demarcation between mental and physical illness" (Jones, 1993: 127). A new medical terminology was adopted such as hospital, nurse, patient and so on, because these were deemed to be less stigmatizing, and by 1934, almost all hospitals had a program of activities. Different associations that had been initiated amalgamated at the outbreak of the Second World War to become the Mental Health Emergency Committee. In 1946, this became the National Association for Mental Health, now known as MIND.

In the USA, from 1900 to 1940, social services, previously provided by religious organizations or religious volunteers, were slowly taken over by federal and state governments. By the mid-1960s, the role that religious organizations had played in helping the needy, including mentally ill persons, had become almost entirely replaced by government programs (Koenig, 2005).

These two chapters bring to a close my research of the historical development of Christian theological understanding of insanity and developing attitudes of Christian lay people and ordained persons during the same period. The chapters were presented so that I could place my current investigation within the context of historical Christian comprehension. Although other authors have previously detailed the information, this is the first time that these works have all been brought together in such a manner.

Some important issues covered still have implications for today. For example, concern of those who commit suicide; humanity and impaired rationality; and that the devised ritual of exorcism, while not occupying the same position as in earlier centuries, is still performed in the twenty-first century.

In the next chapter, I present evidence of Christian involvement and ministry today where there is mental ill health. How apparent is Christian care?

Chapter 4

Christian activities in contemporary society concerning people with mental illnesses

Interest surrounding mentally deranged people has, according to Pattison (1986), invariably had some place of concern either by the churches or individuals. Mental disorder, he feels, has always been looked on as an evil contrary to the wishes of God, which is the reason for it provoking, as it should today, a response within the Christian community.

There is evidence of a Christian response in contemporary society. Boutwood (2003) brings attention to Foskett's sentiments that there used to be great silence in the area of mental health, religion and spirituality; but that this is beginning to change. In the early 1980s, according to Boutwood, there were only lone voices bringing attention to the basic human and spiritual needs of people with mental health disorders, but now there is much activity.

Religious developments

There have been theological, liturgical, and spiritual developments in the twentieth century.

For example, an earlier part of this study recorded that, in historical Christian times, people who committed suicide were not buried in consecrated ground. Today, Christian persons who take their own lives when mentally ill, are afforded the same religious rites in passing as other Christians, but entrenched attitudes take a long time to change. So even today, it is believed important to correct misunderstanding on the issue of victims of suicide and their salvation in the Christian

Church. For example, Rolheiser (2003), a Roman Catholic priest who regularly writes for the *Catholic Herald*, feels that each year he needs to write on the subject of suicide because of the misconceptions surrounding it. There are those, he maintains, who still appear to understand suicide as the ultimate act of despair, although he believes there are, increasingly, signs of change. He advocates that the Christian response to suicide should not be one of horror but to understand it for what it is, a sickness, and to cease misgivings about that person's eternal salvation because of it.

Theological dialogue had been misconstrued down the centuries regarding what constitutes a human being and its relation to mental disorder. This led to misinterpretations about whether persons with these disorders, when irrational, were fundamentally human beings to be treated as such. Despite eventual belief that persons with mental illnesses were fully human in spite of impaired rationality, it seems that contemporary society feels a need by Christians to reinforce this. For example, Sentamu (Building Partnerships, 2004) emphasizes that mentally ill people do not loose their essential humanity, and asks everyone to recognize this, and that health and social services should respond accordingly.

Although the notion of demonic possession waned over the centuries, there is still apparently some belief in evil spirits and the use of exorcism today. According to Batty (2002), the Church of England's Deliverance Ministry, set up in 1974, has teams of clergy and psychiatrists in each diocese and investigates every year dozens of claims relating to haunting, poltergeists and demonic possession. The head of the Deliverance Ministry in Worcester sees deliverance as an alternative form of therapy for people who have strong religious beliefs. Batty reports of a recent survey by the Mental Health Foundation where several respondents had voiced their concerns about the practice of exorcism, and most of these felt it was damaging to their mental health. However, a consultant psychiatrist, who had treated many people after deliverance, believed that exorcism did not of itself cause much mental illness. He felt that it could be beneficial for the Church and the psychiatric profession to work together when someone had spiritual beliefs.

Freidli (2000), Mentality's chief executive, raises the same point that stories of demon possession in the New Testament continue to cause problems within Christian churches, particularly where there is a sense of failure to distinguish between evil and mental ill-health. Likewise, Lerner agrees that "the belief that mental illness is a medical, as opposed to spiritual, condition is, in historical terms, a quite recent phenomenon, and psychiatry's religious roots, as well as mystical attitudes toward the mentally ill, linger even in contemporary times" (Lerner, 1997: 145-146).

An observation by Littlewood and Lipsedge (1995) that in the rest of Europe, unlike in the UK, many societies carried out similar religious healing ceremonies for both physical and emotional distress and do not make this country's customary separation between the two, needs clarifying. It is a fact that, according to my experience, in the UK today where Healing Services take place, there is a practice to invite those who are ill to be anointed regardless of whether there is mental, psychological or physical sickness.

Intercessory prayer has already been cited earlier in this study as a means of seeking healing in the earlier centuries, and this continues today. Mary, the Mother of

Jesus, has been held in high esteem down the centuries by Christians and is prayed to, under the many titles given her, for comfort and consolation. A devotion that has sprung up, in the twentieth century, is one to Mary, under the title of Our Lady of Mental Peace. In 1956, Catholic chaplains at the Metropolitan State Hospital in Massachusetts decided to promote the position of Mary in Mental Health. An outcome of this was devotion to Mary under the title of Our Lady of Mental Peace. In 1963, Cardinal Cushing of Boston, a great supporter of mentally ill people, dedicated a twelve-foot statue of Our Lady of Mental Peace at the hospital. Both Pope Paul VI and Pope John XXIII blest the medal portraying the image. The devotion has since spread to the UK, New Zealand and Australia. This kind of devotion is not that of expecting a cure, but for spiritual uplifting in the midst of sorrow and despair whatever the cause or degree of mental disorder.

Research

The focus on people with mental illnesses, since emptying of the asylums, has led to more awareness of them in the community, partly through media attention, and often in traumatic circumstances. There has been a growing realization by some Christian individuals that people with mental illnesses have needs that are not being addressed, and this has led to research work undertaken by interested parties.

Koenig gives results from a survey, of a sample of almost a hundred hospitalized men, carried out in the USA between 1987 and 1989, on the relationship between the use of religion as a coping behavior, and depression. The only characteristic that predicted lower rates of depression was the extent to which patients relied on their religious faith to cope. Results from another survey, in the late 1980s, of four hundred persons, show that those who attended church at least once a week were approximately half as likely to be depressed as those who attended church less frequently, and this was true regardless of age, sex, race, level of social support and degree of physical illness or functional disability. Another report, concerning the relationship between religious coping and self-esteem, "found that persons who relied heavily on religion to cope had very high levels of self-esteem" (Koenig, 1997: 61). Koenig adds that some of the most powerful evidence for religion's positive effects on mental health comes from studies that have successfully used religious interventions to treat emotional disorders.

Hammaker (1998) gives the outcome of a multi-perspective survey undertaken in Alaska, in the 1990s, of mental-health consumer needs that affirms the importance of faith communities. The third phase of the survey produced a survey return of three hundred and thirteen questionnaires that showed that fifty percent of the stakeholders in the Alaska mental-health system constituting practitioners, administrators, families, and consumers, (consumers being those with mental health disorders), identified participation in church or religious activities as important. Hammaker states that perhaps the most encouraging result of this study is that there is clearly the potential, for all those with interest in the mental-health system and the church community, to proceed together to coordinate their efforts to assist in support of people with mental illnesses and their families. However, he feels that the publicly supported mental health service system has a tradition of very infrequently using church-based resources for its clients. Hammaker suggests that, for many people with mental illnesses, church and religious activities may be a considerable potential resource within the range of supports needed for psychiatric rehabilitation.

In the USA, Nooney and Woodrum (2002) built on recent research, using the 1998 General Social Survey. They consider the findings to be significant for clergy, lay people, and others concerned with personal and institutional religious impacts on mental health. The study assessed religious coping and church-based social support as mechanisms explaining religious benefits to mental health. Nooney and Woodrum advocate that it would be helpful for persons seeking to improve the beneficial effects of religion at institutional level to consider the ways church membership and attendance can pose hardships. Since negative interaction was found to be a significant predictor of depression, ways need to be developed to reduce undue demands on, and criticism of, vulnerable church members. Nooney and Woodrum suggest it would be productive to develop ways of reducing the strong impact of negative religious coping, and to express traumatic experiences within a positive religious outlook.

Ellison and Levin (1998) identify that research studies in America, in several fields, have markedly increased interest in the complex relationship between religion and mental and physical health. Part of their brief was reviewing some of the research of the religion-health connection. They found evidence of mental health benefits of religion among women and men and of different ages and from various socioeconomic classes and geographical locations. They discovered documentation of the wholesome effects of a variety of social resources on mental and physical outcomes. Religious communities are often channels for various sorts of social support; and compassion and kindness, especially towards the less fortunate, are theological imperatives in most major religious traditions. Experiences of volunteering and assisting others can benefit both parties. Small groups sometimes engendered by churches and synagogues may foster a sense of community that can lead to individual members feeling loved, cared for, valued and integrated. Various aspects of religious involvement may promote better health by enhancing feelings of self-esteem or intrinsic moral self-worth. By developing a close personal relationship with a divine other who loves and cares unconditionally each individual, persons may gain a sense of self-worth. Alongside solace gained through private religious activities, persons receive help through pastoral counseling as well as though church programs and church sponsored small groups. Existing findings, according to Ellison and Levin, demonstrate that rates of morbidity and mortality in certain religiously defined population groups are, on average, somewhat lower than among non-religious or less religious people.

The Mental Health Foundation (MHF) (2004), a mental health charity, established in 1949, is a United Kingdom organization with main offices in London and Glasgow. The organization uses research and projects to help people survive, recover, and prevent mental health problems. One of its primary goals is to actively reduce the discrimination and stigma that confront people who have mental health disorders. At the forefront of its work is the task of endeavoring to identify the needs of people with mental illnesses. Part of its work includes initiatives in exploring religion, spirituality and mental health. In 1997, the Foundation published *Knowing our own Minds*, a report based on a survey in which over four hundred mental health service users participated. This was a user-led survey on alternative and complementary treatments and therapies in mental health. The follow up research from the *Knowing our own Minds* project was the *Strategies for Living* project (Faulkner and Layzell, 2003), whereby seventy-one people were interviewed in depth. The results showed that religious and spiritual beliefs were often cited as elemental in providing meaning in people's lives, and a few participants named their religious faith as one of the most helpful factors in their lives. The overwhelmingly predominant theme running through the most useful supports mentioned was the role and value of relationships with other people.

Friedli (2000) points out that growing interest in religion/spirituality, and its significance with regard to people with mental illnesses, raises important questions about the role of spirituality in mental health promotion, the relationship between mental health service providers and spiritual leaders, and the attitudes of faith communities to mental health issues. Some important points she raises emerged from the results of the aforementioned survey by the MHF in 1997. These included various aspects of religious involvement that were deemed as helpful, such as that belonging to a religious community is valued through a sharing of beliefs and a sense of community, and that many people with mental health disorders have found great comfort from their religious communities. Equally, the survey revealed that some people had been damaged by their experiences with religious groups.

Foskett (2000) believes that one of the major fruits of the user/survivor movement has been the work of the MHF. The results of research by people with mental illnesses from the projects *Knowing our own Minds* and *Strategies for Living* were shared at the Alternative Conferences where there was an atmosphere of a fundamental community and of the dignity and ability of service users. Nicholls (2003), Research and Training Co-coordinator for the *Strategies for Living* project at the MHF, reports on further developments from the project. One of the three themes that particularly came up in discussion groups, at the fourth Big Alternative Conference in London in March 2001, was of religious and spiritual beliefs and practices. There was additional evidence for the need of a holistic response, which embraces being sensitive to people's spiritual and religious needs, which is starting to surface from a further project.

Between 2000 and 2002, a user-led research project, supported by the MHF *Strategies for Living* project, was undertaken in Somerset to explore the religious and spiritual resources and needs of some people using mental health services, and their experiences of services and local faith communities. Twenty-seven people were interviewed of which seventeen were women and ten were men of whom the majority were, or had been, Christians. The findings demonstrated that, among those who had been involved with a church or religious group, there were quite contrasting experiences and attitudes. The religious help that was most useful was practical and caring but some participants had felt rejected. Implications included the need for more effective links needing to be built between local and national faith communities and mental health services, and practical help from people in faith communities to be encouraged (Nicholls, 2002a). It was hoped that the results of *The Somerset Spirituality Project* would help people to appreciate how important spirituality is for some people whose experiences covered a spread of mental health disorders (Nicholls, 2002b).

Gray (2001), of Worcester Community Healthcare NHS Trust, reports on a survey undertaken to measure attitudes of members of a congregation. It was conducted at a standard Sunday church service using as a sample, the congregation of sixty-eight people of a predominantly white, middle class, evangelical Anglican community. The congregation was addressed at the beginning of the service with a short explanation and the questionnaire was distributed to all members aged over sixteen. The questions were read out from the front as the forms were completed individually. Two members declined to participate. The results, when compared with those from the general UK population, showed that the church group expressed less negative and rejecting attitudes to people with mental illnesses than the respondents of the general population sample. There was no evidence of judgmental attitudes. The report indicated concern that the church group had major worries about dangerousness and unpredictability and found service users hard to talk to. The conclusion was that further public education opportunities should aim to change damaging negative perceptions of those with mental illnesses.

Swinton (2001b) discusses research based on six in-depth interviews with a purposive sample of three men and three women who had experienced a mental illness for at least two years. He confirms that the inability by others to understand and to accept the reality of their situation was something that was particularly clear in their encounters with church communities, and that the church community was found to be uneducated about mental health problems. He discusses aspects highlighted in the case studies of lack of understanding and various forms of resistance within a congregation. He sees spiritual care as much a way of *being* as a way of *acting* and feels that the resistance sprang from the fact that the congregation was fundamentally uninformed about mental health problems.

Promotion of mental health care/spirituality

Apart from research undertaken attempting to identify the needs of people with mental illnesses and the role of members of faith communities, some organizations and individuals work particularly in promoting religious and theological principles across the spectrum of mental health care, and others include this in a wider agenda.

The Sainsbury Center for Mental Health (SCMH) (2003b) is an example of such work. It is a registered charity, founded in 1985, that aims to influence national policy and encourage good practice in mental health services, thus working to improve the quality of life for people with severe mental health problems. One of its reports, *Forward in Faith* (Sainsbury Center for Mental Health, 2003a), chronicles the development of a pioneering initiative to build bridges between faith communities and mental health services in the London Borough of Newham. The report charts the establishment and progress of Newham's Department of spiritual, religious and cultural care over the last two years. The Department was established following research published in SCMH's report *Keeping Faith* in 1997, and has initially focused on linking people with a mental illness in acute wards to their spiritual communities. Copsey, *Forward in Faith*'s author and leader of the initiative, is a Christian Minister who worked for five years for SCMH and is coordinator for spiritual, religious and cultural care in the Mental Health services of East London. He believes that the experience in Newham is clear evidence that mental health care can only be truly holistic when the religious, spiritual and cultural needs of people are fully taken into account and responded to.

Copsey (2003) and his team of coordinators liaise with the traditional Christian communities. A psychiatric nurse who grew up within a Pentecostal church is forging links with the black community. Other members of his team work with the Asian, the Jewish and the Muslim communities. The aim of his team is to provide, on the hospital wards, a wide range of spiritual resources reflecting the whole community, and to eventually be able to respond spiritual needs whatever belief or faith tradition.

Another example is the Association for Pastoral Care in Mental Health (2004), a national ecumenical movement, founded in 1986 through the pioneering spirit of Christian parents whose son was mentally ill. Its aims are to raise awareness in mental health services and churches of the spiritual needs of people with mental health problems; to change attitudes for the betterment of people with mental illnesses; and to offer a variety of understanding and support. Vallat (1999) defines its aim as to enhance the quality of life, self-respect and spiritual growth of those affected by mental and emotional problems by encouraging in different ways, including that of stimulating church congregations and other faith communities, to be alongside those affected by mental health difficulties. Boutwood (2003) suggests the vision of the Association, that faith communities should be places where people belong, where needs are met, is a real sign that the Presence of God is here.

This Christian-based voluntary Association has individual members and affiliated groups who recognize the importance of spiritual values in mental health. It has a network of supporters throughout the UK, and welcomes and encourages people of whatever faith or belief system. It offers drop-ins, befriending schemes, training courses and awareness-raising seminars and conferences. Its regular newsletter gives publicity to local activities and events that take place around the country with reference to mental health. It gives those with mental illnesses, as well as other interested parties, the opportunity to have their voices heard.

The Bishop John Robinson Fellowship is another organization working in this field. It was established in 1994 at the Bethlem and Maudsley NHS Trust, the Institute of Psychiatry and Heythrop College, University of London, in memory of Bishop John Robinson, and is established within the Spiritual and Pastoral Care Service of the South London and Maudsley NHS Trust. It has a national profile and services a national network among people interested in religion/spirituality and mental health. Its work focuses on the relationship between religion/spirituality and mental health, with the intention of promoting religious and theological principles across the spectrum of mental health care. It has developed three major strands, those of research, education, and information. Its aim is to foster good practice in respect of religion and spiritual factors in mental health care, and to ensure maximum religious and spiritual support for people with mental health needs, their families and carers. Conferences and Forums are arranged through this Fellowship and a platform for discussion and articles is through a newsletter (Bishop John Robinson Fellowship, undated). Head (2002) describes the contents of this newsletter as covering a broad range of people's experiences at the meeting point between religion/spirituality and mental health.

Mentality (2004), founded in 2000, is a new non-governmental organization dedicated to working at mental health promotion and faith, and is affiliated to the

Sainsbury Center for Mental Health, previously documented. Amongst other specific aims, it campaigns to end discrimination against people with mental health problems and to promote human rights and civil liberties. It works alongside and with many local and national statutory bodies and organizations, and targets the general public and many specific groups.

Building Partnerships (2004), another movement, was set up to promote debate and positive action by exploring how London's mental health services and faith communities could work together to improve mental health and mental health care. The report on a Kings Fund workshop, held in early 2001, is the first briefing in a planned series of briefings and workshops. This particular workshop concentrated on working with Christian churches whose congregations included a large number of people from black and ethnic minorities. People from these churches as well as people working in mental health services participated in the workshop. Many people related that their personal experiences of religion and spirituality were central to their lives and at the heart of how they handled and coped with their mental distress. Black church communities can play an important role in advancing understanding and how mental health services can help churches to support people with mental health problems, through building new and effective partnerships.

Lowther (2004), medical advisor to the Salvation Army International Headquarters, reports on a groundbreaking international workshop under the banner of the MMA HealthServe, Mobilising Christian Healthcare Mission organization. The Overseas Health Care Advisory Forum of the Churches' Commission on Mission and the Evangelical Missionary Alliance jointly ran the workshop. There were eighty-eight participants, fifty-two of whom were overseas nationals. Simms, one of the workshop's contributors, having reviewed the changes in practice and advances in treatment, believes it is more important than ever for Christians to provide the care and treatment of people with mental illnesses, and this he feels would need efforts to alter attitudes inside and outside the Church. Lowther concludes that every person is challenged to mediate God's presence to this unfortunate group of human beings.

Resources

As awareness of the need for understanding and support of people with mental illnesses, their carers and families has increased, other sources of communication have been initiated and used to expand that awareness. Over the last years, a number of resources have emerged that are educational and informative and contain suggestions on ways of doing this.

The long running quarterly magazine *Way of Life* of The Guild of Health, within the Church's Ministry of Healing, includes reports on conferences, details of guild groups carrying out their ministry of intercession, book reviews, and information of forthcoming events associated with the ministry of healing. There is also a web site that offers anyone keying in to it the chance to ask for prayers for themselves or others (Holmes, 2002).

A resource pack *Traveling Together.... Towards Mental Health* was published in the early nineties by the Southwark Anglican Diocese Board For Social Responsibility Mental Health Working Group (Southwark Diocese Board, 1992). The resource pack was the outcome of a very informative and challenging Diocesan Synod debate, in 1992, about the care of people with mental health problems. Hall, Bishop of Woolwich and Chair for Social Responsibility, feels a sense of urgent concern that the resource pack should be very widely used.

In 1994, the National Schizophrenia Fellowship held the first of four conferences on religion and mental illness. The conferences addressed the need for training and raising awareness of mental health issues among religious leaders. This initiative had come about because of the realization that a significant number of people with mental health problems turn to churches and other religious groups for support. The end product from this initiative was a booklet, *Promoting Mental Health: The Role of Faith Communities, Jewish and Christian Perspectives* (Health Education Authority, 1999), published in the hope that it would prove a valuable resource for anyone striving to promote mental health within their faith communities.

Coping with... Mental Illness (Truscott, 1995) is a response by the Church. The booklet contains insights regarding causes of mental health, and is an attempt to enlighten members of Christian communities.

An ecumenical group, convened by the Newcastle Diocesan Board for Mission and Social Responsibility in 1996, produced a resource pack *I am not an* Illness (Newcastle Diocesan Board, 1996). Allen, of the Trust Chaplaincy Center at St. Nicholas hospital, Newcastle, believes that those who suffer mental illnesses in society today are often stigmatized because of the fear and prejudice of other people. He reminds readers that the tormented individual in the New Testament story of "Legion" (Mk. 5:1-20) was a social outcast until Jesus treated him as a person. Although the public's response was uncertain, Jesus insists that the restoration of the individual's health was bound up with his return to family and friends. Allen feels that all have something to offer to one another in becoming more fully human and, in this spirit, the resource pack is offered to the churches.

The Carers Christian Fellowship (2004) was launched in 1997 to give support to people caring for relatives or friends. The support is mainly through a quarterly newsletter, the contents of which are often supplied by the carers' own contributions of poems, reflections and letters. Carers are linked up where this is desired and some meet together in local groups. Quiet Days and Fellowship Days are held, and personal support is offered by letter or by telephone. This support is for any carer including those who are looking after people with mental illnesses.

In the USA are further examples. For instance, according to Koenig, Pathways to Promise, an Interfaith Organization in America, "is considered 'the' national resource center for religious groups needing education, advocacy, or other services that address severe and persistent mental illness" (Koenig, 2005: 188). Fourteen faith groups and mental health organizations founded this organization in 1987 with the aim of facilitating the faith community's work in reaching out to those with mental illnesses and their families (Pathways to Promise, 1999). Its website includes details of videos such as Ministry and Mental Illness, Creating Caring Congregations (Closed-captioned), and Mental Illness and Families of Faith. Also available are booklets, pamphlets, and brochures reaching across different denominations. The website is described by Koenig as an incredible source for information about severe mental illness.

Pastoral Care of the Mentally Ill: A Handbook for Pastors (Davis, 2000), published in the USA, is another example of a resource for pastors, Christian education leaders, and other interested ministers. It advises what to do and what not to do when ministering pastoral care to people with mental illnesses, told through stories of people suffering such illnesses.

One of many publications in America offering guidance in this area of pastoral care is *Caring for the Soul R'fuat HaNefesh: A Mental Health Resource and Study Guide* (Address, 2003). It is edited by Address who hopes that congregations do something to reduce the stigma of mental illness and raise the awareness of mental health issues within congregations and communities. The guide is for use by both lay and professional leadership, and the content can be adapted to any denomination.

In the UK, there are further examples. *With a little help from my Friends... Working together for mental health* is a video initiated by members of the Association For Pastoral Care In Mental Health. It is meant for ordinary people to help them reach out in friendship to those with mental health problems. It attempts to address the fear and ignorance that can leave people with mental illnesses and their carers feeling isolated or rejected. The video demonstrates how friends can make an enormous difference by giving just a little of their time (Association For Pastoral Care, 1996).

Another illustration by way of communicating is the use of a leaflet, for example, *Dementia – who cares?* The Social Welfare Committee of the Catholic Bishops' Conference of England and Wales (Social Welfare Committee, 2000) produced this leaflet for circulation in parishes and pastoral centers. This leaflet is specifically directed towards those caring for people with dementia or working pastorally with them, but the content could be applied to carers of people experiencing other mental illnesses. The information given focuses on the spiritual needs of these people and on the needs of those who care for them. It asks for information, formulated in questions, as to how parishes can be of help in these circumstances. A number of appropriate passages are given from scripture as well as some useful addresses/contacts (Social Welfare Committee, 2000). More recently, the Marriage and Family Life Project Office (2006) of the Catholic Bishops' Conference of England and Wales has produced a series of leaflets available on the Internet. These include one on mental health and pastoral care. *What is life like if you or someone in your family has a mental health problem? ... and what can your parish family do to make a difference?* It covers three areas: home-centered care, parish-centered care, and community-focused care. There are suggested scripture readings, help-lines, websites and resources for support and advice.

A modern means of communicating is by use of the Internet. The Church of England Guilford Diocese (2004), on their website, offers a guide on attitudes and the authors admitted having to face the reality of deeply ingrained prejudice against disabled people, when drawing it up. The biggest handicap encountered by people, is the attitudes of others and this included the authors themselves. The readers are invited to reflect on the needs of carers in congregations and the attitudes towards people with mental health problems. A recommendation is that members of church congregations should be reminded regularly of how important it is to use descriptive language and ideas that do not belittle or exclude people, for example, using "mentally ill" which depersonalizes people. The guide refers to discrimination and stigma being very common experiences for people with mental health needs and that fear is the general attitude towards mental health. This fear is perpetuated and reinforced by the predominantly negative and sometimes inaccurate media portrayal of mental health issues. The guide recommends supporters or befrienders to help and that the Church follow Christ's example by providing emotional and practical support.

Carers and people with mental illnesses, because of their experiences and needs, have initiated the establishment of pastoral self-help support groups. For example, in 1994, at St. Mary's Roman Catholic Cathedral in Newcastle, a meeting was called inviting carers and friends to come together to voice their concerns. This came about because I had questioned publicly how much pastoral and spiritual support was available, and known to be available to those experiencing a mental illness and to their families (Hunneysett, 1994). Following from this, awareness days were held involving carers, clergy, mental health chaplains and other mental health workers. Themes included raising awareness amongst the churches and training for clergy. The need for the church's liturgy to reflect the experiences and hopes of both sufferers and carers in a realistic way was highlighted, and the value of an opportunity for carers to come together for mutual support was also seen as important. An outcome was that carers began meeting once a month for support and quiet reflection and prayer.

An offshoot from this meeting in Newcastle was an Open Meeting held in Middlesbrough later the same year. A pastoral support group for carers of people with mental illnesses, that had tentatively started, was firmly established as an outcome of this meeting. The monthly meetings include prayer as well as listening and sharing. People with mental illnesses alongside carers and friends have participated in these meetings.

A mental health pastoral support group was inaugurated in 2000 in a Catholic parish in Glasgow. Those who attend appreciate the spiritual support through shared prayer and the coming together for mutual support and for information. A weekly pastoral support group for people experiencing mental illnesses began in 2006 in Middlesbrough. Participants benefit from sharing in prayer, reflection, and listening in a confidential, non-judgmental atmosphere, in a small group setting.

There are retreat centers scattered around the country that focus on supporting carers. Many retreat houses offer quiet breaks and while these do not specify carers of those with mental illnesses, some are particularly focused towards concern for carers. For example, in Stockport there is a non-residential Shalom Center that runs a Care for the Carers scheme known as Oasis for Carers, on behalf of Sisters of Charity of Our Lady of Evron. In Penmaenmawr, Wales, the Noddfa Center, also known as Noddfa-Caring for Carers, is a retreat center with residential accommodation. Carers are particularly welcome with Short Breaks for Carers, and Carers' retreats are offered. Hexthorpe Manor in Doncaster has particular concern for caring professionals and home carers and the persons that they look after. It offers special provision including residential accommodation for both carer and person cared for, to come together. Holy Rood House, Center for Health and Pastoral Care, in Thirsk, has a holistic and therapeutic approach and offers residential accommodation (Retreat Association, 2002). Carisbrooke Priory, in association with the Acorn Christian Healing Trust, is a non-residential Center for Christian Healing and Wholeness on the Isle of Wight, and has particular concern for those suffering with mental and/or emotional distress.

Christian counselors are available and many carers of people with mental illnesses avail themselves of the service they offer. Those with the illnesses may also access this support. For example, the Association of Christian Counselors (ACC) (2004), founded in 1992, is described as a catalyst for excellence in Christian care and counseling. It includes, in its vision, the provision of a nationwide system for the recognition of training in Christian counseling and pastoral care. A body representing Christian counselors develops relations with institutions, such as the social services and health authorities, and with denominations and professional bodies. It publishes a quarterly journal *Accord*, the contents of which include book reviews, articles, prayers, letters, details of courses, and forthcoming conferences.

Likewise, in the USA, is the American Association of Christian Counselors (AACC). Koenig (2005) notes that it is clearly the largest and best known of the Christian counseling national associations in America. Their quarterly magazine, *Christian Counseling Today*, has a wide circulation.

Another example is the American Association of Pastoral Counselors (AAPC) (2004), founded in 1963. It is an interfaith organization representing more than ninety faith groups, and affirms, as a moral imperative, that mental and emotional illness must be embraced on the same basis and to the same degree as physical illness. A Gallup Poll, conducted in the early nineties, showed that sixty-six percent of the respondents preferred a professional counselor who represented spiritual values and beliefs, and eighty-one per cent preferred to have their own values and beliefs integrated into the counseling process. Pastoral counseling is a major provider of mental health services in the USA. The training possesses a depth that reaches far beyond that of many other mental health professionals of the core disciplines and its discipline maintains the natural connection between the physical, mental, and spiritual dimensions. It is recognized across the mental health field that this connection cultivates a firm and lasting base for treatment of the whole person. Pastoral counselors provide clinically accountable and spiritually sensitive care to those who turn to them for help. Koenig (2005) notes that in order to be certified, AAPC also requires endorsement by one's faith community.

Availability of specifically Christian Homes for people with mental illnesses was hard to determine, but I was able to locate one locally. The Mulroy Nursing Home, described as a Care Specialists for the Adult Mentally Ill, is located on the outskirts of Middlesbrough. The owner/manager is a committed Catholic Christian and full-time nurse at the Home. The focus is on each individual as a human being entitled to be treated with dignity and respect and with needs catered for.

The nursing profession

There has been renewed interest amongst the medical profession on the perspective of spirituality within the nursing profession, which interested parties believe could have profound influence on attitudes towards people with mental illnesses.

A debate on spirituality was conducted recently in the *Nursing Times*. Wright (1997), one of the instigators of this, was amazed at the huge response it provoked. This reaffirmed his belief, that judging from letters received, there is a deep and unsatisfied hunger among many nurses, and patients and others, to explore and open up the spiritual dimension of nursing practice. For example, one of the respondents, Emdon (1997), is adamant that it is the spirituality that makes nurses human and that it is in being human that makes them good nurses. Hall (1997) responded by recalling her experience of watching midwives who gave care with skill and love, and she realized that they had the ability to reach beyond the practicalities, and were able to give spiritual care. Bennett (1997) concluded that Christianity would always lead to the greatest physician of all, Christ.

Moving into the forum specifically of nursing and mental health care, McKie and Swinton discuss what they perceive to be the serious neglect of the "classical" virtues in ethical reflection upon mental health nursing. If an ethic focuses on abstract principles to the exclusion of character and the significance of community, it will inevitably fall short in delivering fully person-centered care. Human virtue enables people to fulfill their function appropriate to their status as human beings and it is these virtues that enable a mental health nurse to function well. Themes from the psychiatric nursing tradition as in care, personal relationships, alleviation of suffering, and the complexity of the human being, have corresponding virtues. McKie and Swinton see as important, that rather than questioning what the mental health nurse should be doing in particular circumstances, virtue ethics asks what kind of person should the mental health nurse be, in a particular situation, in order to make the right decisions. For example, friendship is one of a number of virtues that allows the nurse to venture into areas of relational development and therapeutic possibility by incorporating everyday issues. This enables the "primary focus to remain on the patient as a *person* rather than the patient as a *problem*" (McKie and Swinton, 2000: 39).

Nolan and Crawford (1997) argue that some of those most in need of spiritual care are people experiencing a mental illness or some psychological distress. They explore why they feel that mental health nurses need to appreciate the nature of spiritual well being. The authors believe that the language of spirituality provides a way of talking about meaning and purpose, and they feel strongly that recognition of the spiritual dimension of nursing will enable practitioners to accept the beliefs and values that patients hold. Nurses will then start to understand the meaning that those who are ill attribute to life. This will lead into beginning to comprehend the nature of their suffering, a means by which they can commence sharing the humanity of their clients because it is through this sharing of their humanity that, Nolan and Crawford believe, healing is initiated.

Just as the previous report advocates mental health nurses understanding the nature of spiritual wellbeing, so too, Swinton and Kettles (1997) discuss the nature of spirituality as a therapeutic part of nursing care. They argue that a person's spirituality is the overarching framework within which a person interprets and makes sense of who they are. When individuals become defined by their prognosis, the possibility of stereotyping and stigmatizing become very real. For example, instead of suffering from schizophrenia, a person becomes a schizophrenic. Stereotypes have many associations as in this case being dangerous, and importantly in this discussion, only thought of as being capable of distorted spirituality. Swinton and Kettles feel there should be an approach that accepts and respects the individual as a whole person with physical, emotional and spiritual needs. They believe that a person's spirituality offers hope, meaning and a purposeful frame, and taking into account a person's spirituality makes it possible to redefine an individual as a person to be cared for rather than as a problem to be dealt with.

Although a number of research projects in this chapter have already been reported, it seemed more appropriate to link this account, because it relates to training of nurses, with this section rather than the earlier one. Dring, a qualified nurse, reports the results of research he carried out after his disappointment at not receiving any teaching on religion and spirituality during his four-year training course. He believes that spirituality is the root of human experience, and without any doubt relevant to psychiatric nursing where patients may be probing for the meaning and purpose of their lives. Data was gathered from forty students undertaking the Diploma of Higher Education Nursing Studies Mental Health Branch. Dring concludes from the results of the questionnaire and interviews of respondents, that in the course of their nurse education program, spirituality was not sufficiently covered. He hopes that this will be addressed in the near future so that "nurses are better prepared to fulfill an important part of their role, that of spiritual care giver" (Dring, 2000: 7).

In conclusion, McSherry (2000) suggests it could be argued that nursing today emerged out of the ethos of the Judeo-Christian principle of charity, and he believes that if nursing fails to bring back the spiritual dimension to the center of its work, then the profession is in danger of being replaced by something dehumanizing and cold.

This all looks very promising but much of the survey demonstrates local responses and local initiatives. It is difficult to discern how far this awareness raising, campaigning, and support, penetrates Christian congregations at grass roots level where the outcome of understanding would be expected to be visible in attitudes and action. In a later chapter, I will report on a survey of attitudes in Christian congregations towards people with mental illnesses.

Meanwhile, having looked specifically at Christian activities and support, I decided to explore contemporary attitudes in society before comparing attitudes of the general public with those of Christian congregations. I present my investigation into contemporary attitudes in the next chapter. What is the extent of concern about people with mental illnesses in contemporary society?

Chapter 5

Contemporary attitudes of the general public towards people with mental illnesses

People with mental illnesses were of limited concern to the general public before their de-institutionalization in the late 1960s and early 1970s.

Borinstein (1992), reporting a major research project in America, explains that previously the study of public attitudes toward mental illnesses and people experiencing the illnesses were mostly the concern of the mental health professionals. Mental illness was a private matter between the family and the medical profession. This changed with de-institutionalization and the problems associated with the implementation of community-based mental health care. Mental illness was brought into the public sphere, and what had been hidden had become a more visible social concern. Consequently, issues of mental illness may have become demystified but had become more complex, and there was apprehension as to how the public would respond.

In contemporary society there is concern by some of its members about people with mental illnesses and the associated stigma. Crisp (1999) observes that records of ill people being stigmatized go back centuries especially of people with mental disorders, and he agrees with Borinstein (1992) that the general public has, for a century or more, been shielded from people with mental illnesses by the presence of mental hospitals. With the closure of the asylums, and the emphasis on care in the community, the general public is more aware that those with mental health disorders are living in the community, the neighborhood, and possibly even next door, and as a result, public concern has been increasing.

Research

This increased awareness of people with mental disorders being in the community, and concern by interested parties, has instigated research on attitudes towards them.

Most research projects are administered by professional bodies and executed in society at large. However, more recently, service users have initiated and activated surveys. There is a cautionary note in *Making It Happen*, a guide to delivering mental health promotion, produced by Mentality, that there are discrepancies between data on public attitudes to mental health and the experiences of people with mental health problems (Mentality, 2001). Some possible explanatory reasons can be given for this. Byrne (2001), whose principal research interest is the stigma of mental illness, suggests that, while surveys carried out in society identify levels of awareness, belief systems, fears, and stereotypes of these disorders, those of the public who are not affected or who are disinterested may decide not to take part, and others may give the sociable desirable responses.

In 1998, the Royal College of Psychiatrists started a five-year campaign entitled *Changing Minds: Every Family in the Land* with the aim of reducing the stigma attached to mental illnesses. In order to guide the campaign, the campaign management committee, chaired by Crisp, commissioned the Office for National Statistics (ONS) Omnibus to carry out a survey to determine opinions of the British adult population relating to people with mental illnesses. One thousand, seven hundred and thirty-seven people participated in the survey and results showed that negative opinions about mental disorder were prevalent, a quarter of the respondents agreed to statements that people with severe depression are a danger to others, and people with schizophrenia were generally seen as unpredictable and dangerous. The conclusions were that negative opinions indiscriminately over-emphasize social handicaps which can accompany mental disorders, thus contributing to the social isolation, distress and difficulties in employment that people with mental illnesses encountered (Crisp *et al*, 2001).

Government departments also use the Research Surveys of Great Britain (RSGB) Omnibus to carry out a weekly survey of two thousand adults, aged sixteen and over, conducted face-to-face in-home throughout Great Britain. The surveys have included a series of statements about mental illness, covering a range of issues from attitudes towards people with the illness to opinions on services for them. The annual surveys serve as a tracking mechanism, and the results of the 2000 survey are of particular interest to this study.

Very briefly, the report of the survey, conducted in 1997, showed that the vast majority of respondents had a caring and sympathetic viewpoint and the perceptions the public had of mental illness were quite positive. There was concern over levels of responsibility that might be given to people with mental illnesses, of coming into contact with them, and of integration of them into the community. However, there was sympathy with regard to services being provided for them (Department of Health, 1997).

The results of the 2000 survey were similar to the results of the 1997 survey. Between eighty-three and ninety-four percent had a caring and sympathetic view towards people with mental illnesses. The public's perception of mental illness itself was quite positive with ninety-two percent believing that anyone could develop a mental illness. However, only sixty-six percent disagreed that one of the main causes was lack of discipline and willpower. There was a more positive attitude on how much responsibility should be given to people with mental health problems, but only in comparison to the results of 1997. For example, twenty-four percent believed that anyone with a history of mental health problems should be excluded from taking public office, a decrease of eight percent.

Further results showed that the questions about coming into contact with people with mental health disorders demonstrated a greater acceptance than of the 1997 survey. However, this again was only of a comparative measure. For example, the highest percentage responding favorably to any of the six statements about coming into contact was forty-nine percent and the lowest percentage was nineteen percent. Support for integration of people with mental health problems into the community also appeared to be growing, but in two of four instances, less than fifty percent were favorably inclined. Attitudes towards available services were discussed and results indicated support and sympathy for people with mental illnesses, but again, only in comparison with the 1997 results. In two instances of three, less than fifty percent showed positive attitudes (Department of Health, 2003a).

Key findings of the 2003 survey showed that attitudes had worsened slightly between 2000 and 2003. Although the summary report of the results showed that the vast majority of respondents had a caring and sympathetic attitude, percentages of those who agreed that society has a responsibility to provide the best possible care had decreased by five percent to eighty-nine percent. Younger respondents tended to adopt a slightly less tolerant attitude. There was little change in public perceptions of mental illness itself and about the levels of responsibility that possibly should be given to people with mental health disorders. Older people tended to be more in favor of restrictions on people with mental illnesses, particularly of them taking public office.

A new statement was introduced into the 2003 survey that "People with mental health problems should have the same right to a job a anyone else." Sixty-seven percent agreed to this, with females slightly more in favor than the males. The results showed that levels of fear and intolerance of people with mental illnesses have tended to increase since the surveys began in 1993, and that there was some evidence of an increase over time in fear of people with the illnesses. However, there were no significant changes from 2000 on questions about integrating people with mental illness into the community (Department of Health, 2003b).

A project conducted on behalf of the National Association for Mental Health (MIND) in 1998, as part of its three year *Respect* campaign, was the largest UK inquiry into social exclusion and mental health ever undertaken. It was conducted to try to discover the extent and the nature of the social exclusion experienced by people with mental health problems in Britain today, by listening to views of mental health service users, mental health service workers, and general employers, and providers of goods and services. A panel of experts was brought together to consider evidence from hundreds of individuals, groups, and organizations. The panel received strong evidence of the discrimination that people experience as a direct result of their illnesses, and that it occurs in every aspect of life (Health Matters, 2003).

Dunn, a freelance writer and editorial consultant specializing in health and social care issues, details the results of the Inquiry in *Creating Accepting Communities*. She notes that according to already existing research, there is accumulating evidence of the discrimination experienced by people with mental illnesses in Britain, and the outcome of which is their systematic exclusion from society. While the more recent Community Care policies have changed the place of health and social services for people with mental illnesses, the ethos of segregation that underpinned mass institutionalization has not, according to Dunn, disappeared. This is mainly because the barriers in the old institutions have been replaced by economic and social barriers within the community which, although less obvious, are just as effective. Once people have mental illnesses, access to finance, work, social networks and secure homes become harder and as a result, "many of the most vulnerable people in Britain today are caught in a spiral of social exclusion that is almost impossible to break" (Dunn, 1999: 10).

To see if these results of attitudes of the general public and those connected to the mental health services coincided with the opinions of those with the actual illnesses, results of a user-led survey were examined. This survey originated out of a meeting between Muijen, the Director of the Sainsbury Center for Mental Health, and service users because, at that meeting, the participants had recalled appalling events that had personally happened to them in the wider community. The project was coordinated and conducted by users of mental health services, and one of the aims of the survey was to find out from users themselves how they perceived the actions and attitudes of the public towards them. Fifty-eight of the seventy-six respondents were contacted at two separate day centers in London. A further eighteen users were interviewed by their key workers. The survey deliberately targeted people with enduring mental ill health who had been in contact with the mental health services over a long period of time. A series of semi-structured interviews was carried out. Respondents were asked questions about a range of community groups and individuals with which they might have contact, for example, friends, the Department of Health and Social Services, Housing departments and agents, the police, community organizations, neighbors, local communities, religious organizations and churches, work, and family.

Rose (1996), a senior researcher at the Sainsbury Center for Mental Health and herself a service user, details the results in *Living in the Community*. The results showed that sixty-one percent of the public was unsympathetic and twenty-six percent were indifferent to people with mental ill health. People with severe mental illnesses perceived considerable prejudice and stigma in the community. Many experienced contacts as negative and rejecting, with examples of demeaning behavior, avoidance and hostility. When dealing directly with agencies such as housing and benefits, they felt that they were at the bottom of the pile and discriminated against when compared to other users of such agencies. Although not a universal condemnation, the majority found contact with these agencies to be both demeaning and stigmatizing. The most frequently cited reasons for the negative attitudes that surfaced were fear, ignorance, lack of contact with people with mental health problems, and negative media portrayals. The majority of those who were in contact with their churches were positive about this, referring to their personal and social side of their experiences at church as well as the religious ones. These results demonstrated that users perceived the negative attitude that the general public had towards them. In answer to her question as to whether or not the community cares, Rose observes, from the results of the user-led survey, that people are still far removed from being able to understand or welcome people with mental illness into their neighborhoods, and that the majority of people with mental health problems feel that the community does not care.

In the USA, research has also revealed attitudes of discrimination, for example, with regard to housing. In this instance, two third year medical students, Alisky and Iczkowski of St Louis, Missouri, highlighted specifically concrete attitudes of prejudice in the results of their research carried out in 1988. They were looking at community behavior towards mentally ill people with regard to accommodation. The research investigated the availability of public housing in the city and county of St Louis, and the willingness of landlords of private housing to make available houses to rent, to psychiatric patients. Twenty-two percent of the managers contacted refused to rent to a mental health patient or denied that a vacancy existed. Twenty-two percent would have nothing to do with mentally ill people no matter what the economics. That finding was a barometer of how patients were accepted in a large metropolitan area with the conclusion that people with mental illnesses have to deal with not only the burden of their illness but also significant barriers to housing, that they "are shut out of public housing by lack of available units and out of private apartments by high rents and outright discrimination" (Alisky and Iczkowski, 1990: 95).

This attitude of discrimination with regard to housing manifests itself in neighborhood opposition, including "not in my back yard" (NIMBY) campaigns, an outcome of the impact of provision of mental health services. An editorial in the *British Medical Journal* affirms that the NIMBY attitude is universal, and that worldwide, the initial community responses to community care have not been positive (Sussman, 1997).

Address (2003) reports that in the USA, approximately twenty to twenty-five percent of the single adult homeless population, suffer from some form of severe and persistent mental illness, and that it is estimated approximately one-third of the homeless in major Canadian cities suffer from a mental illness.

In America, the NIMBY phenomenon was evident from research undertaken in 1989 on behalf of the Robert Wood Johnson Foundation Program on Chronic Mental Illness. It was a survey, by telephone, of one thousand, three hundred and twenty-six individuals as representative of adults aged twenty-one and over. Although there was lack of negative attitudes about people with mental illnesses, nearly half of the respondents would not be pleased to have mental health facilities in their neighborhood, implying that "the NIMBY phenomenon may exist as a real barrier to opportunities for people with mental illness" (Borinstein, 1992: 192).

In the UK, a project took place between 1988 and 1992 before and after people with mental illnesses were moved from large psychiatric hospitals into community-based mental health facilities in North London. The study was an attempt to discern public attitudes towards the decision to close psychiatric hospitals, and to identify the needs of the public before patients moved into their neighborhood. A study and a control group of residents were interviewed before and after patients moved into a mental health facility in their neighborhood. The study consisted of a hundred immediate neighbors of patients being moved from a long-stay hospital ward. The control group comprised a hundred residents of a road parallel to that of the study group. No significant differences in responses were found in relation to cultural and educational background, age or sex. While most of the respondents were in favor of opening mental health facilities in their area, the results appeared to suggest that the public perceived mentally ill people as different and in need of hospital protection. A NIMBY attitude was revealed whereby the local residents considered people with mental illnesses as least positive neighbors, and indicated that they would rent accommodation to people with other illnesses such as diabetes, epilepsy, and learning disabilities, but not to those with mental illnesses (Reda, 1995).

Kaminski and Harty (1999) were the coordinators of a Mental Health Awareness project early in the nineties based in Kirkintilloch, a semi-rural area to the North of Glasgow. They also found that not only was the quality of life of people with mental illnesses adversely affected because of their illness, but also by the rejection of their fellow people, and they reported that previous research showed that the NIMBY attitude continues to exist.

Several witnesses in the *Creating Accepting Communities* report nimbyism as perhaps one of the "most graphic and brutal manifestations of social exclusion." Dunn (1999) reports that NIMBY campaigns continue to disrupt the provision of community mental health facilities. It is not only the local inhabitants who waged NIMBY campaigns, but witnesses inferred that local councilors and politicians are often guilty themselves of discriminatory attitudes.

Contributory factors to negative attitudes

A number of themes, for example, fear, ignorance and lack of contact, have emerged from the research behind the negative attitudes that have surfaced.

Fear is highlighted in a number of surveys and searches. For instance, Rose (1996) briefly refers to two previous studies, one of which was by MIND in 1994, that had looked at the attitudes and opinions of a thousand adults and the other, by Levey and Howells in 1995, that focused specifically on perceptions by the public of people with schizophrenia. Of the first, over fifty percent of the people questioned were concerned about risk to the public from dangerous mental health patients, and the results of the second were even less optimistic, demonstrating that both these studies revealed a high level of anxiety regarding behavior of mentally ill people. The results of the user-led project showed that sixty-seven percent of the respondents believed that the general public was afraid of people with a mental health disorder and a further twenty-two percent thought that they sometimes were. This meant that almost ninety percent of users perceived the public to be afraid of people with mental illnesses, evidence that people experiencing these illnesses, using the mental health services, have to carry the added stress of being aware that they are a source of fear for those around them.

Hayward and Bright (1997) summarize the main findings of research done in the fifties, sixties, and seventies. These earlier projects concluded in general that the public feared and disliked people with mental illnesses and wished to avoid them at all costs. In their current review of surveys, the authors offered four possible explanations to the root cause of the unfavorable view of mental illness, the most straightforward one being the "dangerousness" idea, that people fear mentally ill people because they believe them to be prone to violence. Reda reports, with reference to the project referred to earlier on moving patients from large psychiatric hospitals into community-based mental health facilities in North London, that the majority of respondents regarded social factors as a main cause of mental illness and mentally ill people were associated with "violence, physical assault, difficult communication or bizarre behavior" (Reda, 1995: 732).

In order to characterize current public conceptions related to recognition of mental illnesses and perceived causes, dangerousness, and desired social distance, Link *et al* (1999) used the USA General Social Survey data involving one thousand, four hundred and forty-four respondents. A strong connection was discovered between mental disorders and perceived likelihood of violence. Sussman (1997) believes that fear continues to obstruct moves towards caring more humanely for mentally ill people in the community even though many of these fears are unfounded, and others could be lessened by sensible policy making.

Another theme behind the negative attitudes that has emerged from the study is that of ignorance. For example, of a survey undertaken in 1989 of approximately one thousand, three hundred and twenty-six respondents in America, the results showed that twenty-five percent said that they were not well informed about mental illness, and sixty percent felt they should know a good deal more about it (Borinstein, 1992).

In London, a research project of two hundred fifteen participants revealed that many, who admitted to being fearful of people with mental illnesses, were afraid because they did not know much about mental illness (Wolff *et al*, 1996a). The survey project in London referred to by Reda gave evidence that, although the participators could not distinguish between mental illness and mental handicap, they showed sympathy towards the term "mental handicap" which was expressed "by their willingness to donate money to charitable organizations for the mental handicapped only" (Reda, 1995: 731).

There was evidence from the results of the previously mentioned ONS survey of one thousand, seven hundred and thirty-seven adults, of the belief that people with mental illnesses could pull themselves together. There was also widespread opinion that it was difficult to converse with mentally ill people, that their behavior was unpredictable, and that people with mental illnesses actually felt differently. This was likely to account for some of the social distancing and isolation that people with mental disorders experience and, as a consequence, a continuation of lack of familiarity of the realities of what those with mental illnesses undergo (Crisp *et al*, 2001).

The Nuffield Council on Bioethics (2003) is an independent body, established by the trustees of the Nuffield Foundation in 1991, to consider the ethical issues arising from development in medicine and biology. Recently, it produced its dossier *Mental disorders and genetics* (1998) that took two years of research. It believes that stigma mainly results, not from encountering difficult behavior that those with mental illnesses sometimes displayed, but from ignorance and misconceptions about mental disorders. Hayward and Bright (1997) also reported, in their review and critique of literature, an attitude amongst the public of a belief by lay people that mentally ill people chose to behave as they do

Behind negative attitudes, a third theme that emerged was lack of contact although there were conflicting views on this. On the one hand, responses by respondents of the survey of the seventy-six user participants gave lack of contact with people with mental health problems as one of the most frequently cited reasons believed to account for the negative attitudes towards them. A conclusion was drawn that if the general public were able to identify their common humanity with mentally ill people, they were likely to be more favorably disposed towards them (Rose, 1996). Hayward and Bright (1997) also reported that some studies showed that contact with people with mental illnesses increased positive attitudes. Research has shown that if prior contact with someone with a mental illness has already been made, there is less stigma and fear of danger (Warner, 2001).

On the other hand, Reda (1995), referred to earlier with regard to NIMBY attitudes, concluded from the research that contact with mentally ill people was not enough to change public perceptions of mental illness. According to Crisp *et al* (2001), even if some respondents knew of someone with a mental illness, this apparently made no difference with regard to negative attitudes when the illness was schizophrenia. For Sussman (1997), it is a dilemma either way because he suggests that it is possible that if the public is presented with much improved patients, they may see them as the exceptions, but if they are presented with the stereotyped typical patients, there may be a change of attitudes or a risk of reinforcing the stereotype.

Influences

Having looked at some contributory factors to negative attitudes, I now turn to possible influences on these attitudes. The literature survey revealed that the media and the medical profession are, at times, influential in exacerbating negative attitudes towards people with mental illnesses.

The style in which the media manifests mental illness was demonstrated in the results of a study that the Media Group at Glasgow University began in 1992. Five hundred and sixty-two items of press coverage were sampled, and in general, the category of violence to others was by far the most common, outweighing the next most common, that of a sympathetic approach, by a ratio of almost four to one. Items linking mental illness and violence tended to receive prominent treatment while sympathetic items were largely designated to the letters, the problem page, or health columns. Another part of the research was an audience reception study involving seventy people. In writing their stories, the audience groups demonstrated a remarkable ability to reproduce the media style and language. Forty percent of people sampled believed serious mental illness was associated with violence, giving the media as the source of their beliefs. There were very few positive images portrayed in the media showing that people can recover, achieve, or be active in their own right. The results showed clear links between media portrayals and attitudes of the general public to policies such as community care (Philo, 1994).

A study conducted in London in previous years found that ordinary people had similar views as those represented by the media on psychiatry in its over-inclusion of portrayal of people with mental health disorders being dangerous and having unpredictable behavior (O'Grady, 1996). The opinions given about violent behavior in the ONS survey, already mentioned, may have been influenced by dramatic coverage of violence by the media at the time the survey was conducted, more than by personal contact. If this is so, then Crisp *et al* (2001) propose that any de-stigmatizing campaign needs to pay attention to reporting by the media.

Service users have strong views on media representation. For example, more than a half of those who took part in the user-led project thought that the media could improve its portrayal of mental illness (Rose, 1996). The results in *Creating Accepting Communities* revealed that many individuals, who use or have used psychiatric services, felt that that the media was prominent in fashioning and reinforcing the fear and prejudiced reactions that people have to those with mental health disorders, that it has great power in inventing and perpetuating biased attitudes towards mental health service users, and that the opinions of service users themselves were rarely heard in mainstream media. Discriminating attitudes have been made worse in recent years by sensationalist media coverage of violent crimes committed by people with mental health problems, and this kind of reporting, misguidedly and damagingly links mental ill health with a tendency to violence. The consequence of this link was that the media has been complicit in worsening biased attitudes towards mental health service users, and thereby directly advancing their social exclusion. This, in turn, gives the opportunity for feigned justification for driving people with mental health disorders to the very edges of society (Dunn, 1999).

Byrne (2000) reiterates negative portrayal by the media. He believes that by giving narrowly focused stories based on stereotypes of people with mental illnesses, the media perpetuates stigma, and Haghighat (2001) makes the point that exposure of many positive contacts can be undone by a handful of salient news items on a murder of a person by someone with a mental illness. Warner (2001) too, feels strongly that media exaggeration, biased reporting, and unfavorable attitudes among the general public, continue to be significant problems.

Apart from the media, the literature survey revealed that the medical profession has influence on attitudes, but Byrne (2000) holds that, even though stigma of mental disorders has existed long before psychiatry, the psychiatric profession in many instances has not helped in reducing either stereotyping or discriminatory practices. Dunn (1999) believes that a psychiatric diagnosis can be the onset of a process of social exclusion instead of leading to a therapeutic or support process, and she feels that this process is triggered off partly because of the nature of psychiatric services, which are, according to Dunn, experienced as ghettoized and stigmatizing. Chaplin (2000) likewise thinks that the work of psychiatry can be powerfully stigmatizing and this includes the unpleasant side effects visible to the public of prescribed medication. Furthermore, a Mental Health Act assessment at a patient's residence can be a cause of tremendous stigma to the patient and family because of the visible services involved such as police and ambulance. This suggests that Mental Health Acts assessments have the potential to be the most stigmatizing event that any family with a member with a mental illness will undergo.

McKay (2000) questions how the general public can have a rational approach to people with schizophrenia when learned journals display advertisements that promote a product through negative stereotyping, this with reference to a negative implication in one of the top psychiatric journals concerning a person with schizophrenia. He feels that professionals like himself should be prepared to examine their own beliefs about serious mental illnesses before trying to change attitudes in society at large. Being associated with mentally ill people taints the Agencies that serve them, according to Warner, and mental health professionals sometimes are known to hold attitudes towards mentally ill patients that are similar to those of the general public; "they may even be *more* rejecting" (Warner, 2001: 455). Even with reference to the concept of shame as an experience of mental illness, Byrne (2000) holds that professionals are no different in this regard as they conceal mental disorders in themselves or in a family member.

Stigma

The literature survey has disclosed a number of contributing factors and influences of negative attitudes towards people with mental illnesses, but another word with negative connotations frequently mentioned in relation to mental illness is "stigma."

Definitions in a dictionary of the word "stigma" include "a mark of infamy," "any special mark," "a disgrace or reproach attached to a person," and "a scar." More detailed explanations can include a mark upon the skin by burning with a hot iron as a token of infamy or subjection, as in branding; a distinguishing mark or characteristic of a bad or objectionable kind; or a sign of severe censure. The stigmata, from the word "stigma," describes the marks resembling the wounds of the crucified body of Christ, said to be supernaturally impressed upon the bodies of certain saints and other devout persons, but these same wounds were evidence of treatment meted out to a person viewed as an undesirable or criminal, thus a sign of disgrace or condemnation (Editors, 1999: 1624).

Authors contribute to these definitions. For example, Byrne (2000) describes stigma as a sign of disgrace or discredit that sets a person apart from others. Goffman explains that upon meeting a person, evidence can suggest an attribute that makes the person different from others and of a less desirable kind. Thus the person "is reduced in our minds from a whole and usual person to a tainted, discounted one" (Goffman. 1963: 3). Some note that stigma often carries a religious significance, that the afflicted person is viewed as sinful or evil (Kleinman, 1988; Haghighat, 2001). Porter (1998) reasons that placing the sickness apart upholds the fantasy that those without the sickness are whole and, as a result, disease theories can reinforce general moral bias. Kleinman (1988) suggests that it can be seen as a moral connotation of weakness and dishonor which results in the person being defined as someone different, upon whose persona are projected the traits that others regard as opposite to the ones they value. In this sense, stigma helps to define the social identity of the person. The Nuffield Council on Bioethics (1998) reports that mental disorders are often stigmatized and this stigma is a significant and widespread feature of mental illness of which the degree varies in accordance with different disorders, and that assumptions about what is standard, and hence about what differs from standard, will vary over time and according to cultural context. People with mental illnesses, as well as suffering the condition of the illness, often have to suffer the associated stigma.

It is possible that stigma could be to do with cultural influences because Western ideas have always linked morality and virtue with health and reason (Byrne,

2001). This division of standards manifests itself in relation to mental illnesses. Many features of mental disorder are defined in terms of difference or deficiency as compared with a standard defined within a social context. Kleinman (1988) suggests that this difference in the bizarre actions of those who are mentally ill invoke the cultural categories of what is ugly, feared, alien, or inhuman thus breaking the cultural conventions about what is acceptable appearance and behavior. Massow, chair of the *Creating Accepting Communities* Inquiry, found the project revealed that, although those diagnosed had little in common, immediately they were diagnosed, their world changed, not because of their illness but "because they had suddenly been marked *different*," this difference being manifested by discriminatory attitudes (Dunn, 1999: vii). It would seem therefore, that when users described themselves as having been marked *different*, it is their way of expressing stigma, this being different. Goffman (1968) reiterates that the central feature of the stigmatized individual's situation in life is a question of what is often, if vaguely, called "acceptance," that although the stigmatized person belongs to the wider group according to society, meaning he is a normal human being, he is also "different" in some degree. Thus Goffman argues, the painfulness of sudden stigmatization can come "not from the individual's confusion about his identity, but from knowing too well what he has become" (Goffman, 1963: 133). He concludes that, "by definition, of course, we believe the person with stigma is not quite human" (Goffman, 1968: 15).

Another aspect that differentiates people is the labeling factor. In certain societies, the stigma is so powerfully identified with the cultural labeling of the patient's illness that it affects all the person's relationships and may lead to ostracism (Kleinman, 1988). One of the recommendations of the user-led survey, *The Somerset Spirituality Project*, is that it needs to be remembered that being labeled can have very negative effects on people (Nicholls, 2002b). A history or label of mental disorder can lead to stigma in the absence of any behavior that differs from the norm (Nuffield Council on Bioethics, 1998). Hayward and Bright (1997) report from research that labels, such as mental illness and mental patient, carry a negative overtone, and that many findings support the view that a label of psychiatric illness is stigmatizing. The stigma of mental illness is not so much related to a person's appearance, according to Byrne (2000), as to context and is a powerful negative characteristic in any social relations. It is this labeling as mentally ill which carries internally, shame, secrecy and lower self-esteem and externally, social exclusion, discrimination and prejudice (Byrne, 2001).

The *Creating Accepting Communities* Inquiry revealed that discrimination against people with mental health disorders was evident in service provision, education, employment, and in every aspect of life, and the most powerful evidence concerning these issues came from people who had received psychiatric diagnoses such as doctors, health service workers, managers, office workers and teachers (Dunn, 1999). Warner (2001) similarly believes that people with mental illness are subject to prejudice, discrimination and stigma, as does Sussman (1997). Stigma is not a rare event but, according to Corrigan *et al* (2001), stigmas about mental illnesses are widely endorsed by society in general.

Evidence that people with mental illnesses are aware of stigma is identified from the user-led project. The results suggest that where choice was involved, for example, friends, church, or family, the interviewees felt the group on the whole was positive. Where there was no choice as in the Department of Social Security, the police, the neighbors, or the local community, they believed that the group treated their mental illness status in a stigmatizing way. The interviewees felt that the police were particularly prejudiced and contact was especially negative. Consequently many users tried to hide their mental health problems from members of the community and professional organizations because they were afraid of stigma. They felt the stigma strongly and the results showed that it was quite common for people with mental health problems to feel the need to hide this from the community. This sense of a guilty secret was a burden to many users and it seemed to be a direct outcome of discriminating attitudes by the wider community. Although those interviewed differentiated between the positive and negative features of the community, it was the latter which far outweighed the former (Rose, 1996).

Putting aside the user-led research, it is difficult to measure stigma in general surveys, according to Byrne (2001), because people who are prejudiced tend to play down their negative attitudes and alternatively, in real life situations, behavior is difficult to study. Haighighat (2001) discusses the value of attitudinal research questions. He describes the results of his reflections on a unitary theory of stigmatization, as the reinterpretation of stigmatization and reformation of the relevant concepts. He argues that like all attitudes, stigmatization has three components: cognitive, for example, schizophrenics are violent; affective, for example, anxiety; and discriminatory, for example, refusing to give someone accommodation. He suggests, with reference to research, that what is measured by attitudinal questions is cognitive hypotheses and is not a measure of attitudes as these do not contain the other two components. He does believe that cognitions matter in that the inevitable awareness of those who are stigmatized, of the cognitive elements of people's attitudes, puts the former in a position in which they feel vulnerable.

Papadopoulos *et al* (2002) concluded from their research, comparing attitudes by first and second generation Greek Cypriots and those of White-English ethnicity, that stigma surrounding mental illnesses continues to run deep in most societies. There have been numerous studies that highlight that there is a stigma associated with mental illness, according to Kaminski and Hart (1999). An outcome of the project that they coordinated was that the Greater Glasgow Health Board acknowledged the scale of the problem and that the root of it was an attitude problem. The conclusion drawn was that stigma of mental illnesses is reflected in language, in attitudes, and in society, and that from a young age the public are bombarded with imagery that is discriminatory regarding mental illness. As it is society's language and culture, it is therefore society's responsibility.

In the past psychiatrists working in developing countries often noted the low level of stigma that attaches to mental disorder. The World Psychiatric Association Program Against Stigma and Discrimination Because of Schizophrenia identified a number of factors in the developing world that promote greater tolerance and community support for people with serious mental illnesses. These include the absence of large-scale institutional care and the strength of the extended family. However, in parts of the developing world with advancing industrialization and urbanization, evidence now suggests that the stigma of mental illness is increasing (Warner, 2001). On the other hand, Borinstein (1992), working in America, notes that the stigma attached to seeing a psychiatrist has lessened because of greater public awareness. Contrary to this, Address makes reference to an example of the "ignorance and stigma that still need to be overcome in American society;" how an individual has to come to grips with the social stigma once a diagnosis has been made, and maybe even to coping with the great fear of disclosure (Address, 2003: 33).

Possible reasons for stigmatization

A number of reasons for these negative attitudes towards people with mental illnesses in society have been unearthed by research and are explored.

Corrigan *et al* (2001), from research carried out in the USA, report two opposite concepts of attitudes. One is benevolence, that of seeing people with mental illnesses as childlike and in need of watching "by a compassionate caretaker." The other is authoritarianism, the belief that a "paternalistic mental health system" should make decisions for persons with mental health disorders because they cannot care for themselves. Whichever attitude of benevolence and authoritarianism is prevalent, gives rise to avoidance of persons with mental illnesses.

Address (2003) feels that people are set in their ways and often form opinions based on stereotypes. Byrne's (2001) theory is that negative aspects of unpositive stereotypes are a reflection of the negative attitudes of those who stigmatize. Haghighat (2001) develops this concept. Humans beings, although generally not endorsing the misfortunes of others, are willing to use the "unfortunate others" attitude to feel happier about themselves. Thus, those who stigmatize, benefit from the presence of people who feel stigmatized because the latter provides them with psychological dividends, that is, examples of persons they can consider worse than themselves. Research has shown that people with higher intelligence and higher self-esteem would not feel it so necessary to demean people with mental illnesses in order to feel positive about themselves and, therefore, are likely to have more positive attitudes towards them.

Haghighat has suggested another reason for negative attitudes. If people are not responsible for illness, then this means that it could happen to anyone and reassurance is needed to counteract this. Consequently, some might propose that those stigmatized, or their parents, have done something wrong and are being rightly punished for their sins, thus allowing for "the pursuit of psychological self-interest without unbearable guilt" (Haghighat, 2001: 208). He also questions whether it is possible that the fundamental basis of all stigmatization is the pursuit of self-interest and if so, is a protective device for those who stigmatize and mostly unfair on the stigmatized. It could be argued, however, that it is not necessarily self-interest but possible concern for the community that gives rise to this sort of stigmatization.

According to Hayward and Bright (1997), findings suggest that people with mental illnesses do not necessarily fit into the norms of community living, and people are not comfortable in situations in which the normal rules of social interaction do not work smoothly. They deduce, from previous research, three possible root causes apart from disruption of social interaction. Firstly, that of dangerousness because if there is a tendency to violence then people will keep their distance; secondly, attribution of responsibility as in the people themselves being seen as responsible for their condition, their misfortune. Thirdly, there may possibly be more likelihood of stigmatization if the illness is difficult to treat and with a poor prognosis. Findings of other research suggest that, in general, older respondents and those of a lower educational level and social class are less favorable towards mentally ill people. Finally, the Nuffield Council on Bioethics (1998) reports that stigmatizing attitudes display evidence of lack of understanding, sympathy and respect for suffering fellow human beings.

Consequences of stigma
The consequences of mental illnesses in contemporary society are many.

Mentally ill people themselves often accept the stereotype of their own condition (Warner, 2001; Kleinman, 1988), and are acutely aware of the phenomenon of stigmatization (Haghighat, 2001). A person who comes out of a mental hospital has to face the "unwitting acceptance of himself by individuals who are prejudiced against persons of the kind he can be revealed to be" (Goffman, 1968: 53). Byrne (2000), in listing the adverse experiences of stigma, begins with shame because he believes that mental illness is still seen as a sign of weakness, and that the outcome of private and public shame is secrecy. This secrecy acts in turn as an obstacle to means of treatment and, consequently, people experiencing mental illnesses are removed from potential supports. White (1998) endorses this view that the stigma attached to being mentally ill worsens matters by inducing shame, and this results in persons experiencing the illness denying their distress and failing to seek effective help. Many authors counter persons may delay seeking help that in turn means they will not have access to the medication needed (Haghighat, 2001; Nuffield Council on Bioethics, 1998; Link *et al*, 1999) because, in taking the medication, individuals will feel that they are endorsing the idea that they are "mad." Consequently this has a detrimental effect on their wellbeing and possible recovery. These factors are among the afflictions of community psychiatry (Haghighat, 2001).

The results of the ONS survey, carried out in 1998 on behalf of the Royal College of Psychiatrists to assess attitudes to mental illness and how prevalent the stigma within society, are presented in *On your doorstep*. The aim of this project was to look at issues surrounding mental health in the context of community developments, as some communities are more equipped than others to develop, sustain and promote positive mental health. Two community-based organizations in England were focused on. One was Bromley by Bow Center in the Borough of Tower Hamlets that incorporates primary care, and the other was Health First Health Action, a health and welfare advice project in West Earlham on the outskirts of Norwich. Results revealed that people with mental illnesses are significantly subjected to social exclusion, unemployment rates are higher than for any other section of people with disabilities, and the physical health amongst these people is worse than the general population. Consequently, disadvantages from such discriminatory attitudes create a vicious circle, especially when added to the stigma and the social rejection of local communities, and can limit access to both health treatment and justice (ONS Omnibus, 1998).

Many services users, who gave evidence to the Inquiry reported in *Creating Accepting Communities,* felt that their diagnosis made them "non-citizens" with no rights, no credibility, and no redress from either the state, mental health services, or other members of the public. There was consistent evidence of the discrimination people experienced because of their mental health problems. This occurred in every facet of life, and the discrimination combined to make mental health service users vulnerable to extreme social exclusion that further exacerbated their mental health problems. The results showed that people with mental illnesses are amongst the most seriously and regularly excluded groups in British society. The evidence collected by the Inquiry, as late as 1998, confirmed without uncertainty that people with mental health disorders are acutely excluded in society today. This exclusion does not arise from the mental illness but from the assumptions and bias attached to the diagnosis, and this not only by members of the local neighborhood, but also by health and social care professionals (Dunn, 1999). In other words, people with mental illnesses feel stigmatized.

According to the Nuffield Council on Bioethics (1998), stigmatization damages the reputation and sense of self of the sufferer, making mental illness an object of fear, and causes further injury by various discriminatory actions. Medical disorders place a heavy burden on individual sufferers, on those who care for them and on society at large. Partly as a consequence of the pariah status, people with schizophrenia in the developed world lead lives of social isolation with more curtailed social outlets than is usual in society. Approximately thirty-three percent of chronically, mentally ill people have no friends at all (Warner, 2001). Thus, Goffman says, "lacking the salutary feedback of daily social intercourse with others, the self-isolate can become suspicious, depressed, hostile, anxious, and bewildered" (Goffman, 1968: 24). It is because of concerns, such as people with mental illnesses being unpredictable and dangerous, that the sufferers themselves experience isolation and insecurity making their search for help more difficult (Crisp, 1999). Results of the user-led *Strategies for Living* project suggest that people with mental illnesses had to seek out those whom they thought would accepted them and where this failed to take place, society can only reflect and affirm the isolation and social exclusion that results (Faulkner and Layzell, 2003).

Patients with mental illnesses benefit if they not only accept their illness, but also that they feel in control themselves. However, usually accepting the illness means for most, a loss of this sense of self-mastery. Thus, stigma creates a situation where accepting the illness can mean losing the capacity to cope with it (Warner, 2001). Borinstein (1992) concludes that, unless attitudes change, the prospect of enabling people with mental illnesses to have the opportunity to become an accepted part of their local community remains dubious at best.

Effects on families/carers

Authors report that chronic illness almost always holds consequences for the family and other close personal relationships.

For example, Kleinman (1988) holds that the effect can be very serious, and Goffman (1968), that those related to a stigmatized person are obliged to share some of that person's discredit. Others note that serious mental illnesses can lead to broken family networks. Sometimes, the families are seen as tainted with the patient's deviance and may even be blamed for their relative's mental illness. Those afflicted and their relatives feel shame and are a source of avoidance or criticism. Thus, the relatives caring for a patient with a mental illness may also have to cope with the stigma of having a relative with the illness, and suffer exclusion by the wider community (Dunn, 1999; Nuffield Council on Bioethics, 1998). According to Warner (2001), some react by talking to no-one about the illness for years, not even to close friends, and others respond by withdrawing socially. Identification in the *Making It Happen* guide, of groups of vulnerable individuals at risk, includes carers, but there is a question as to whether there is "professional emotional support readily available locally to those caring for others with mental illness" (Mentality, 2001: 85).

Addressing stigma

The survey produced evidence that there is growing awareness in contemporary society that the problem of stigma should be addressed. It revealed a variety of ways and means of doing this.

Sussman (1997) is adamant that those responsible for health must not be oblivious of the responsibility that society has for the treatment of the vulnerable mentally ill. Byrne (2000) raises the point that examination of the achievements of other anti-discrimination movements leaves mental illness stigma as one of the last prejudices. He advocates that far-reaching action within and outside psychiatry is now needed and, although there is no agreed way of measuring stigma, he believes that gauging public opinion on mental illness is pivotal to understanding and lessening it (2001). In its report, the Nuffield Council on Bioethics (1998) points out that both the stigmatization and the harm which it causes need to be addressed but, generally speaking, believes rectifying injury to reputation and sense of self, will be the harder task. Haghighat (2001) promotes the idea that developing a cure for mental illness is likely to reduce stigmatization but it would need to be effective, not just given as rational data but demonstrated as productive.

Every piece of evidence submitted to the *Creating Accepting Communities* Inquiry, in one form or another, was, according to Dunn (1999), grounded in the need to recognize the unquestionable and equal value of every person, and the ethical bedrock of any challenge to the social exclusion of people with mental health disorders is the recognition of the definite worth of the individual human being. In the *Making It Happen* guide, it is advocated that the needs of the whole person, are addressed and this firstly means treating people as individuals, not illnesses (Mentality, 2001).

The user-designed and led *Strategies for Living* project, already referred to in the previous chapter, was an in-depth qualitative investigation into the supports and strategies that people experiencing mental health problems or distress found to be helpful in their lives. The role and value of different relationships was frequently a means of achieving self-acceptance (Faulkner, 2003), and the information from the interviews conducted showed that the stigma and discrimination people experienced in relation to mental illnesses made the acceptance of others a vital part of their survival strategy (Faulkner and Layzell, 2003).

The outcome of analyses of a study by Corrigan *et al* (2001) in the USA, in which one hundred and fifty-one participants, recruited from twenty-four Illinois community colleges, completed measures of prejudice toward, social distance from, and familiarity with people with mental illnesses, suggested that prejudicial attitudes have direct influence on discriminatory behavior and therefore, changing attitudes may lead to improvements.

Findings also showed that familiarity with mental illness may lessen prejudice towards people experiencing the illnesses, that people who are more aware of people with mental illnesses, through experience of family members or peers or learning at school, are not as likely to uphold prejudicial attitudes about such people and consequently, education and contact programs that promote familiarity with mental illnesses may lessen prejudicial attitudes. White (1998) recorded results of research that showed exposure to be probably more effective than education.

The survey revealed other ideas and thoughts on how to reduce stigma. Haghighat (2001) believes that the public's fear and anxiety as a component of stigmatization, can either be desensitized through contact with patients or relieved through dialogue, thus not a purely cognitive enterprise but one that is likely to arouse more emotion and possibly have some positive effect. He suggests that a forum needs to be provided where people can discuss their anxieties and fears concerning people with mental illnesses, and describes linguistic intervention aimed at engaging people in a discourse of value as a means of promoting shifts in attitudes, an opportunity to challenge whoever has a stigmatizing attitude, and invite whoever might be sympathetic enough to join those who wish to lessen stigmatization. He also advocates a sensible policy to help lessen other fears.

There is evidence that communities can play a major part in addressing stigma associated with people with mental illnesses. Dunn (1999) reports that most witnesses to the *Creating Accepting Communities* Inquiry agreed that mainstreaming was fundamental to social inclusion as they felt that making separate facilities for people with mental health problems, in education, employment or other areas of society, were counter-productive and exclusionary. Advice in the *Making It Happen* guide is to use settings where national and local policies can be joined. It gives the work place as an example, such as linking in with local policies on a return to work following mental health problems, and employing people who experience ongoing mental health problems. It also gives examples of programs to increase employment of people with mental health problems, and suggests that an increase in mental health literacy across all sectors as an important goal in terms of reducing stigma (Mentality, 2001). The Nuffield Council on Bioethics (1998) stress that it is important that access to employment and other opportunities should be based on a person's merits at the time, and not on what might happen in the future.

Following in this vein, a journal, *A Life in the Day*, enables opportunities for presentation and reflection upon new kinds of daytime opportunities that promote active involvement for people who are mental health service users, and is especially committed to giving service users a platform. Grove, the editor, reports a noticeable difference occurring because of the user employment program at South West London and St. George's NHS Trust. It is not just that there is now a number of staff employed who have a history of severe mental illness, but also that twenty-five percent of those applying to the trust are now prepared to acknowledge a history of mental illness. He believes this shows that if the barriers facing people who have become excluded are dealt with, this can sometimes be "the catalyst for a more general rethink about the culture and values of the places where we live and work" (Grove, 2002: p4).

Results from the *On your doorstep* project, referred to earlier, showed that the two community based organizations targeted had a specific organizational culture with definite characteristics. A list of these positive key themes included being uniquely placed to act as go-betweens and having a clear concern with community inclusiveness. A number of stories demonstrated the potential of such organizations to alter perceptions, raise awareness and to educate in areas of need such as where there are severe mental health disorders. The positive and informal involvement of local community groups in situations of this kind made it possible for them to encourage a more educated understanding of emotionally charged subjects, such as mental illness, than would otherwise be possible. It was felt from these results that community organizations could offer a new dimension to mental health services in the way of thinking through new ways of collaboration, and of putting them into practice (ONS Omnibus, 1998).

A further revelation from the literature survey was the possibility that the medical profession has a role to play in addressing stigmatizing attitudes. For example, Crisp *et al* (2001) believe that professionals should listen to patients in order to foster good communications, and learn about their patients as people with individual concerns and needs. In order to achieve this, staff should be sympathetic, and receive adequate training and sufficient time. Moreover, White (1998) suggests that Health Care professionals (including those within mental health) should correct their own stigmatizing attitudes, and he gives, as an instance, that the person should always be separated from the illness by speaking about a "person with schizophrenia" rather than a "schizophrenic." This factor of self-assessment is reiterated by Crisp (1999) who advocates that if stigmatization of mental disorders is to be successfully combated, or if society at large is to achieve this, the medical profession must put their own house in order to start with. Likewise, according to Dunn (1999), although it is vital that mental health service providers acknowledge and support inclusion work outside their traditional boundaries, it is equally clear that the lead responsibility to promote social inclusion for people with mental health problems must be with mental health services themselves. However, Porter (1998) is convinced that if the stigma from mental illness is going to be eradicated, the task cannot simply be left to the doctors.

The education field is another area that has possibilities for addressing the stigma surrounding mental illnesses and relevant issues. For instance, Wolff *et al* (1996a) conducted a study in 1993 on attitudes to mental illnesses of residents in two streets prior to the opening of group homes for people with mental illness. From the interviews conducted, there appeared to be a link between a lack of knowledge and negative attitudes towards people with mental illnesses. People from the lower socio-economic groups, those least educated, those with children, and people from ethnic minorities were the ones who had the most negative attitudes towards mentally ill people.

As the general public is increasingly coming into contact with people with mental illnesses because of the shift to care in the community, Wolff *et al* (1996b) believe that attitudes towards them in communities will play a major role on whether people with mental illnesses will be accepted and socially integrated. They were, therefore, interested in conducting a further study to test the hypotheses that negative attitudes towards these people may be fuelled by lack of knowledge. Two hundred and fifteen people were interviewed. The results supported their hypotheses, especially amongst older people, but negative attitudes among people with children were not necessarily related to lack of knowledge.

Wolff *et al* (1996c) presented a third paper relating to education. They reported that previous research by the Team for the Assessment of Psychiatric Services (TAPS) had shown that only a small number of patients make social contact with ordinary members of the public and this included their neighbors. In order to improve social integration of patients, they felt it was important to discover ways of adding to their number of social contacts within the general public and of sustaining such relationships. It was obvious to them that attitudes of the general public would have had bearing on this. Therefore, to improve the social integration of those with mental health disorders, the Team carried out a controlled study to research the effect of a public education campaign on community attitudes to mentally ill people. This was initiated, firstly, by conducting a consensus of neighborhood attitudes towards people with mental illnesses in urban areas situated in the London borough of Lambeth before the opening of supported houses for such people. After the two facilities were opened in 1993 in staffed houses in this local area, one of the two areas was then targeted with an educational campaign. Following this, the attitude survey was repeated in both areas, and the social contact the patients had with their neighbors was recorded.

The results showed that respondents exposed to the educational part of the campaign showed only a small increase in knowledge concerning mental illnesses. However, there was a lessening of fearful and rejecting attitudes in the experimental area but not in the control area. These were manifested in the attitudes of the neighbors in the experimental area as being more likely to make social contact with both staff and patients.

Also, the patients in the experimental area made contact, and some friendships, with neighbors, whereas those in the control area did not. While there was no significant difference between increase in knowledge in the two areas over time, there was a non-significant trend toward an advance in knowledge in the experimental area, when only the neighbors who had participated in the educational campaign were compared with those in the control area. The authors concluded that, while the campaign did not bring about significant changes in knowledge, attitudes improved, and the social integration of patients was enhanced.

Moreover, when looking at the categories of fear and exclusion, social control or goodwill, the results showed that there was only an overall decrease in the category of fear and exclusion in the experimental area at the follow-up compared to the control area, but the results showed an increase in acceptance of patients in the experimental area. In conclusion, what the Team discovered was that the education campaign did not in itself lead directly to less fearful attitudes but contact with patients did, and therefore, they felt that it is likely that the campaign was effective indirectly on overall attitudes by encouraging contact with the patients.

Other literary research showed that education was thought to be a necessary way to improve attitudes. Hayward and Bright (1997) in their review and critique, agree that there are divergent opinions as to how the issue of stigma should be addressed and mixed opinions on methods of education, but believe that some form of public education would be most useful on a wider social level. Recommendations arising from results of the user-led project *Living in the Community,* home in on the need for education and training (Rose, 1996). Byrne (2000) believes that while there are many different groups of those who stigmatize across society, the starting point for all groups to be targeted, at whatever level, is education. At the least, Haghighat (2001) sees that educational campaigns are likely to be effective in challenging the attitudes of those who stigmatize, of proposing alternative attitudes, and of emphasizing the presence of anti-stigmatization pressure groups and stakeholders. Papadopoulos, *et al* (2002) found, from the results of their research, that knowledge about mental illness was associated with a favorable attitude towards people with mental illnesses, and that aggressive educational campaigns specifically for minority communities are required to confront the stigma attached to mental illnesses. According to Dunn (1999), public education about mental health problems, and mental health promotion, need to be given a much higher profile than they have in the past. She feels that there is a need for sustained and strategic initiatives in order to change attitudes so as to tackle the stigma presently attached to mental health service users.

The Nuffield Council on Bioethics (1998) summarizes that it is very difficult to wipe out stigma, and that there is apparently no easy way, single organization, or piece of legislation, that can eliminate the harm and injury done by the stigma of mental disorder. It will take long-term changes in public understanding of, and support for, those with mental health disorders, to improve matters.

Promotion of positive attitudes

While surveys revealed negative public attitudes, they also demonstrated a substantial amount of good will towards mentally ill people (Warner, 2001), and means of promoting and increasing this goodwill were discovered in the literature survey.

Although the surveys have demonstrated that education is vital to reducing stigma, Crisp *et al* (2001) reason that stigmatizing opinions are not necessarily related to knowledge, and to lessen stigma requires more than increased knowledge of mental illnesses. They point to the concept of protection against discrimination that recognizes that there are those who are different in ways from the majority and that some have disabilities, but this minority has equal rights.

Another perception in reports from the *Creating Accepting Communities* Inquiry is that there is little knowledge or understanding of mental health issues in many schools, colleges, or universities, and that educational bodies do not know how to access advice. For instance, students with mental health disorders may undergo their problems periodically, but may experience discrimination by being prevented, after recovery, from picking up where they left off, because of the structure of many courses, and the necessity to complete within limited time frames. It is suggested that it is especially important to create support systems for people with mental health problems in further and higher education because this can often be when people first experience mental health problems (Dunn, 1999).

With regard to raising awareness in schools, there is some evidence that user-led programs, which are interactive and enable the students to openly verbalize their fears and anxieties, can be effective in changing attitudes. It has been proved that the outcome of pilot programs in schools is an increased knowledge about mental health issues among pupils, and a reduction of stigmatizing beliefs about mental health disorders and those who experience them. There is good evidence to support the effectiveness of peer education (Mentality, 2001). Crisp *et al* (2001) advocate that an important place for any anti-stigma campaign should be in schools because a recent survey indicated that stigma was no less prevalent among young people.

User-led research is the kind that aims to be inclusive by involving mental health service users and survivors because, as they are people with experience of mental health problems (or mental distress), users have their own expertise (Blazdell, 2003). This expertise is frequently passed over by the people involved in planning mental health services. However, more has been done in research projects in recent years in involving people who have, or are experiencing, mental illnesses, to encourage insight into what they feel and want rather than others deciding for them (Faulkner and Layzell, 2003). Rose (1996) insists that users must be given the means to talk directly to the community, perhaps also to hear their side of the story, because she believes that only when this genuine dialogue gets underway that deep-seated prejudice will begin to disappear. Users are quick to praise the mental health services, treatments and personnel when they are considered to be good practice, and the good examples revealed by user-led research can be of benefit to all involved in mental health services (Blazdell, 2003).

Another means of increasing positive attitudes is the work of many trusts and organizations to de-stigmatize mental illness by means of promoting good practice, and there has been a wealth of work undertaken in the field of mental health promotion over the past five years, the *Making It Happen* guide produced by Mentality (2001) being an example of this. A *Defeat Depression Campaign* took place from 1991 to 1996, an activity of the Royal College of Psychiatrists in association with the Royal College of General Practitioners during which time samples of the general public were surveyed three times, the latest in June 1997. A positive attitude change was achieved during the *Campaign*, although there was still space for improvement in some aspects (Paykel *et al*, 1998). Other specific undertakings mentioned already are the National Association for Mental Health (MIND)'s three-year campaign, *Respect,* in the late 1990s, and the Royal College of Psychiatrists' five-year campaign that began in 1998 entitled *Changing Minds: Every Family in the Land*, to reduce the stigma of mental illness.

Examples of good practice include Tees and North East Yorkshire NHS Trust (2002), a specialist Mental Health and Learning Disability Trust that is committed to addressing stigma. In 2002, the Trust secured the *One in Four* exhibition that the Government's *Mind Out For Mental Health* campaign had commissioned, and it was shown at three venues across the Trust region. A growing list of volunteers *Passionate Friends* has been drawn up by the Trust that includes people experienced in mental health such as carers, and those they care for. The volunteers are called on to speak and share their experiences in schools and colleges especially where there are Health and Social Care departments. In 2003, the Trust launched *Open Up*, a long-term campaign to tackle the stigma often attached to mental health problems and, in 2004, secured the national *MindOut* for mental health's new *Headspace* exhibition for display that features photographs of well known musicians and pop stars along with their views and experiences of mental illnesses. Tees and North East Yorkshire NHS Trust (2003) has developed *The Way Ahead*, a strategic direction to stimulate change and develop excellence in mental health and learning disability service with more than a hundred users and carers consulted on the Trust's *Advance* project to modernize services.

Under North Tees NHS Primary Care Trust, a Consortium of Specialist Health Promotion Services in Tees, Durham and Darlington offers a course Certificate in Promoting Mental Well-Being accredited at level three by the Open College Network, North Tees PCT Health Promotion Service. The program is aimed at professionals, and individuals with an interest in mental health and those working with or caring for people who have experienced mental health problems (Tees, Durham and Darlington, 2004).

Some organizations working in this field to promote positive attitudes have been detailed earlier in this chapter or in previous chapters. These include the Mental Health Foundation, the Sainsbury Center for Mental Health, Mentality, the National Association for Mental Health, and the Maudsley Hospital which is part of the South London and Maudsley NHS Trust that works with the Institute of Psychiatry and runs a clinical Pastoral Education Program of which some participants are trainee clergy.

Other recent organizations founded to support and promote positive attitudes include Making Space (Community-Care, 2004), founded in 1982, which provides services across the north of England to carers and individuals affected by severe mental illnesses. It specifically helps those with schizophrenia and their families and aims to promote development of community care facilities and to advance public understanding of the nature of schizophrenia. It offers a number of supports including providing self-help groups and organizing courses and conferences. Another is *SANE* (SANE, 2004), established in 1986, the aims of which are to raise awareness and respect for people experiencing mental illnesses and for their families. It strives to improve education and training and secure better services and offers a national telephone help line, *SANELINE*, set up in 1992. It has its own magazine *Sanetalk* (SANE, 1996) that gives a voice to people with mental illnesses and carers and other interested parties.

An example of a magazine, as an initiative that can help promote positive attitudes, is *Breakthrough*, founded in the mid 1990s and published by Patient Power. It is a national bi-monthly magazine produced entirely by sufferers and survivors of mental illnesses and emotional distress, and carers, and it particularly wants to promote their voices through written material. Its aims include educating, informing and opening up lines of communication between service users and the professional caring services (Marx, 1995). Another example is the charity, Mental Health Matters that began in the 1980s as the Northern Schizophrenia Fellowship, and in 1997, published the first edition of its newsletter *Families and Friends* (Mental Health Matters, 1997). This aims to address issues directly related to carers of people with mental illnesses and to provide a forum for the exchange of ideas.

A further factor that can promote goodwill is the media and although the media appears to have done a good deal of damage, Dunn (1999) believes that it has potential to do a great deal of good. She feels that the excluding behavior of both institutions and individuals is widespread, often running alongside fear and ignorance and not only needs tackling with both education and legislation but also with concerted and strategic use of the media. Recommendations from the user-led *Strategies for Living* project, already detailed, include the government and health education and health promotion agencies supporting the promotion of positive images of people living with mental health problems both locally and nationally, through a comprehensive anti-discrimination campaign (Faulkner and Layzell, 2003). The media were employed to advantage, during the *Defeat Depression Campaign* of 1991 to 1996, to help educate the public about stigma and depression. During the campaign, there was considerable increase in media activities that included newspaper and magazine articles, television and radio programs and interviews on depression. There were acknowledgements by media figures of their own depression. Other media activities employed were press conferences, production of leaflets, and fact sheets in ethnic minority languages, audiocassettes, a self-help video and two books (Paykel *et al*, 1998).

Media incorporates a whole range of communication channels. For instance, according to Haghighat (2001), like all attitudes, stigmatization has three components, one of which is affective, for example, anxiety. To work on the affective component would take works of art, novels or films that are more likely to act on feelings of the public at large. Warner (2001) offers the examples of the story highlighted in Eastenders and the film Shine that conveyed several stigma-busting messages. Modern communication technology offers the possibility of a more successful assault on stigma in schizophrenia than previously. The World Psychiatric Association is taking on board these approaches in a new world wide educational campaign.

Rogers (1996) cites communication as having a key role in every form of medicine and health especially in deciding whether medical research and health programs that seek to administer research-based knowledge are effective in helping to solve health problems. Pozner (2002) advocates the Mental Health Employment Network as it aims to raise the profile of employment for people with mental health disorders and to provide contact among member groups for mutual support, advice, and information, the network's main offering being its newsletter. Byrne (2000) indicates that many positive articles across medical journals and the like are fuelling debate on this issue. He suggests that stigma and its issues should be given a prominent place on the curriculum of all health service professionals and students.

In order to combat discrimination and social exclusion, the *Making It Happen* guide gives a list of possibilities to promote better public understanding about mental health problems that includes firstly, the local media (Mentality, 2001), and Byrne (2000) agrees it will be the media that will be used in any campaign to challenge and replace the stereotypes. Likewise, the Nuffield Council on Bioethics (1998) in making reference to stigma, advocates the need to educate people and combat media representation, as do Hayward and Bright (1997) who believe that a sympathetic presentation of mentally ill people on television and radio, in newspapers, and in the cinema would be useful means of educating the general public.

In America, societal changes such as health and science sections of magazines and newspapers and television programs relating to health, have, according to Borinstein (1992), helped towards demystifying many psychological and mental health issues. When the media and public education campaigns address the issues of fear and exclusion and social control, Sussman (1997) believes it is only then that stigmatization will lessen, and social interaction, and friendships will occur.

These two chapters conclude the report of the survey of contemporary Christian and the general public's attitudes towards people with mental illnesses. Prior to presenting the results of my investigation comparing attitudes of Christian congregations with those of the general public, I decided to explore another area of concern, that of the training of leaders of faith communities. I detail my findings in the next chapter. Will I discover the formation to be adequate with reference to mental illness?

Chapter 6

A survey of pastoral formation of Christian leaders on supporting people with mental illnesses and their families

Priests, pastors, and lay leaders undergo training at institutions founded for the purpose of preparing them for ministry in faith communities. These communities will include those with mental illnesses and their families.

Methodology

My initial intention was to investigate resources used in training for the ministry of pastoral care towards those with mental illnesses and their families. I broadened this to determine whether or not there is a distinctive Christian dimension that priests and ministers bring to this specific ministry.

I limited the sample target to three different ecclesial traditions, the Anglican Church, the Roman Catholic Church, and Pentecostal/Evangelical fellowships, as I deemed it impractical to attempt to collect and analyze data from a wider variety of denominations. The Anglican Church was chosen as the major denomination of the UK. My personal interest is the Roman Catholic Church. The third choice of Evangelical and Pentecostal denomination was because of the different structure and set-up of their faith communities compared with the other two denominations chosen.

I sent investigative letters initially to an Anglican training college and a Roman Catholic training college, each situated within the geographical region to be targeted later, on attitudes in Christian congregations. I explained that I wanted to determine whether there were resources used specifically to train ministers in the field of mental illness, or whether resources for this were included in the general instructions on pastoral care of sick people and their families. If the latter, the quest was for details of the resources and whether mental illness was included. I wrote a similar investigative letter to the Evangelical/Pentecostal leaders of sixteen faith communities situated across the same area. The contact at the Anglican college suggested three further Anglican institutions across England where ordinands are trained. I knew of three other seminaries for the training of Roman Catholic clergy across the country. The initial letters of enquiry were also sent to these six institutions. One of the Evangelical/Pentecostal pastors suggested I contact a training center that he knew of in the UK, and this suggestion was followed through.

I received a number of replies but after examining their content, I felt it was insufficient for the purposes of the investigation. I sent a further letter of enquiry explaining that more specific information was required on training and not just on resources as requested in the first instance. The reason was to try and identify whether there was any distinctive perspective in Christian pastoral formation over and above what would be included in secular training in preparation for care of people with mental illnesses and their families. This letter covered two specific areas. Firstly, it referred to general awareness of people with mental health problems and their care, and listed a number of ways that might be used to help candidates familiarize themselves with the nature of mental illnesses. Secondly, it made reference to a Christian perspective, and asked about the Christian dimension of care that leaders would be expected to perform in the course of their ministry, and the training needed to assist them when embarking on this work.

The second investigative letter was sent to each of the same four Anglican and Roman Catholic institutions previously targeted and the one Evangelical/Pentecostal institution. I made enquiries to Evangelical/Pentecostal leaders for details of other such colleges where training of prospective leaders of their faith communities was undertaken and was given details of another three. I sent to each of these three colleges a copy of the second investigative letter, appropriately modified, as they had not been in receipt of the first one.

Anglican response

Three colleges responded to the first enquiry, and one of these responded to the second enquiry.

One college allocated a two hours training session in its first year, obligatory to all ordinands. The input included reference to mental and psychological illness. Lectures, for example, might have a retired psychiatrist explaining how to recognize the illnesses and how to cope with the situation, how to be effective carers and give effective comfort to families. In the third year, a further session was allocated to issues of pastoral ministry with the possibility of mental illness being included but this session was not compulsory. The college drew on organizations like MIND for information and leaflets. Areas covered include survivors of sexual abuse, marital issues, self-esteem, eating disorders, adolescents, young and old suicides, and gay issues (mental problems). Samaritans and psychiatrists were invited to speak to the ordinands. A number of books were used relevant to pastoral care.

A response from a second college briefly replied that, "this is covered in our regular teaching on issues in pastoral care, which is provided by a senior psychologist. We do not provide specialist courses in mental illness."

The respondent of a third college offered its response as being a "fairly standard reply," and this included the following information.

> *Some people address the issues concerned but usually only a minority. As regards mental illness, there's a course, Clinical Pastoral Education, run through the local mental hospital, which takes six people for an entire term, so it is very intensive. Others will come across mental illness through courses on psychology, counseling, Samaritans, cruse, prison/young offenders. In the C of E system, the assumption, (not always well grounded!), is that more specialist pastoral areas are taught about during training after ordination. We have only two to three years for basic training and that is what it is: basic!*

The one college that replied to the second investigative letter reiterated information already given regarding the clinical pastoral educational course. The college acknowledged that only a tiny percentage of students gained direct access to the basics involved, but that it was done intensively, and that there was feedback from course participants into their college peer group. Less directly connected were several placements in, for example, prisons, and homes for the elderly where many basic issues were raised. This college believed that a significant proportion of students would have some access to mental healthcare even if not concerted. With reference to a Christian perspective, the respondent stated that it required more time than he had to give me. He would be happy to talk "face to face" but not "scramble around in how we do/how we don't address the matters you raise." He added that in the highly complex arrangements of coursework, no one is doing the same thing. Every one is able to address mental health. They take contextual theology seriously as a paradigm for how to meet situations from a practical theological perspective. He concluded that preordination training needs the model of how to do things rather than a checklist of having done superficially more than anyone can possibly take on board (or teach).

Roman Catholic response

Two colleges responded to the first enquiry, and these same two colleges responded to the second enquiry.

The following information was received from one college.

> *We use human resources! By this, I mean we use Catholic psychiatrists, chaplains in mental health hospitals and we have used Stephen Sykes to work with students, explaining attitudes and skills which will help in working with sufferers and their families. I'm sure we don't do enough and your query leads me to think we need to do more.*

The respondent from a second college enclosed a selected bibliography (fifty-eight named) covering disability issues in general and church teaching. He made the following comments.

> *You will note some specific references to mental health issues. Reference is made to the body of*

Catholic social teaching, some of which makes specific mention of disability issues, but the overlying theme of all such documents is the fundamental dignity and rights of the human person.

He enclosed an overview of their BTh degree, indicating that "aspects of mental health care and generic disability issues are covered within the studies on 'Christian Ethics' and 'Social and Health Care Ethics' in particular," and that many of the documents in the selected bibliography would be used within these courses. He added the following information.

Participation in the Clinical Pastoral Education Program run by the South London and Maudsley NHS Trust has recently been introduced into the formation syllabus. For a period of up to twelve weeks, students have the opportunity to engage in full-time clinically supervised chaplaincy work as part of the multidisciplinary team within this Mental Health Care Trust. Students who have undertaken this course have found it very valuable and a useful insight into the needs of people living with mental health issues.

In replying to the second investigative letter, the first respondent reiterated information already given by citing talks, videos, some pastoral placements in mental health care, the use of chaplains working in mental health care settings, and the use of various books (un-named) as resources. As to the specific Christian perspective, the respondent explained that the Christian dimension was always stressed and that "as Disciples of Christ, we hope to encourage our students always (emphasized) to adopt the compassionate, sensitive and listening stance." Hope was expressed that students and priests would have the courage to draw alongside all who were ill and try to understand life from the other's perspective, but that time did not allow for specific training in dealing with mental health problems. While raising awareness was of paramount importance, specific training would be done on-site in hospitals *et cetera.*

The other college enclosed replies from the Director of Studies and the pastoral Director. The Director of Studies replied that formation aimed to give a basic understanding so that students would be able to exercise pastoral care to include prayer, listening, celebration of the sacraments, and support for families, *et cetera.* Most students had some professional experience before entering the seminary and some may have suffered from treatable mental health problems. Some came with a background in medicine, nursing or health care professions. The wide variety of backgrounds of residential students enabled peer formation that might include many aspects of having dealt with mental health either personally, in families, or in working contexts.

He said that the specific area of mental ill health took place in the framework of formation. It was focused on four areas of human formation to include: understanding and prejudices towards persons; spiritual formation to include assisting students to convert attitudes and to form them in the Christian tradition of caring for the sick; intellectual formation to include moral theology and learn that all persons are equal in dignity; and pastoral formation that included workshops and day seminars on an occasional basis to focus on mental illness and problems of mental health. Reference was again made to the clinical pastoral educational program at the Maudsley hospital. The seminary, he said, had access to a school catering for students with special needs and various disabilities and also to another school at which some trainees had engaged in pastoral placements, who then reflected on the experience, both individually and in a facilitated group process.

The Pastoral Director of the same seminary stated, firstly, that my questions did not lend themselves to direct answers; that they cannot train priests to be experts at everything and that there was no programmatic focus on mental illness, no taught course on it. Mental health and psychology were key elements of human and spiritual formation and students would be aware of Christ's outreach to the marginalized and the essential inclusiveness of the Gospel. The policy was to raise awareness of mental health issues through occasional talks and training days. The seminary organized pastoral placements with special schools and psychiatric hospitals that included elements of clinical pastoral education in some instances. While being aware that only a minority of students would do this, others would encounter people with mental illness on more general pastoral placements. Pastoral reflection groups provided a forum for the sharing of experiences and airing of issues, and some students had firsthand experience of mental illness in their family history, through friends, and previous employment. Some would have a background in medicine, nursing (including psychiatric nursing) and social work. A particularly helpful resource was the publication *A Minister's Handbook of Mental Disorders* (1993) by Ciarrotti.

Evangelical/Pentecostal response

Five faith communities and one college responded to the first enquiry, and two other colleges responded to the second enquiry.

Pastoral Care: Mental Health

One of the two leaders of a faith community gave the following information.

> *We don't have any specific training for our folk, or ourselves. We just treat everybody and situation as it comes along. We have dealt with quite a lot of people with mental illness over the years. We are kind, fair and tolerant! It is a bit of a minefield. Christians usually have some patience and I'm sure as we walk with the Lord this will improve. Sorry I don't know of anything specifically we've read which you can use.*

This was followed with a telephone call from one of the leaders in which it was pointed out that, in the New Testament, the fishermen were untrained laymen. He concluded by informing me that they referred to the Holy Spirit as the Holy Spirit Bible School.

A second respondent, a pastor, explained that he was responsible for three churches. At the time of writing, they did not have any program of instruction on pastoral care of sick people and their families.

The following is the response from another pastor.

> *Unfortunately, I am unable to give you any information as regards any resources I have to deal with mental illness; I do not think you will have any more success with any of my A.D.G. fellow ministers. I can say that the A.D.G. Executive have set up a social concerns department which would direct me to various help telephone numbers and seek guidance.*

Yet another pastor replied. He gave the following information.

> *I can only answer from what I believe to be the case in our denomination (Assemblies of God). I am not aware of any specific or general training given to prospective or existing ministers regarding mental illness and the effects on their families. Training in Pastoral Care including those who are sick is given in our Bible College, but most ministers would, like myself, pick up what they know by experience. Obviously this is not a satisfactory situation, but there is only so much that can be covered in a two/three year course where only some students will enter in full time ministry in churches. In addition, there does not seem much written in the Christian press on the issue. Also for some they would see it as the domain of the experts rather than enlightened amateurs.*

He added a final comment that "I trust that your research is fruitful in raising awareness within the Christian Church regarding this issue."

The final communication from the first investigative letter was in the form of e-mail from one of the team leaders who spelt out how the situation was before the arrival of the present leader.

> *It is fair to say that none of the team was formally trained in pastoral care, and their experience was gleaned from their belief in the healing power through the Holy Spirit, years in commerce and, sometimes, specific teaching sessions. We have a firm belief in the miraculous*

and that God can and does heal those struggling with mental problems as well as the physical. As a result, some of the complex cases out of our range ability would be referred for professional help and counsel, usually to Christian contacts/counsel, to assist where more help was needed but not already being provided from other sources e.g. the GP.

He added that the present leader's training at Bible College did not include any specific awareness or input on mental illness. His own year long, part-time course touched on these areas, but not in any depth. There were a variety of scenarios, Ignis Counseling, listening skills, and use of questions that were all embraced and practiced, but he could not remember if recommended reading had been suggested. He felt that those in Leadership in the Salt and Light family of churches were very challenging and presented papers on Pastoral Care from the biblical perspective. He ended with the information that "the church here runs a 'Recovery' course and aims to help people deal (again Biblically) with a wide range of issues in a group setting."

A respondent from a college replied that its courses are aimed at students "who desire to know God more and see God's purpose for their lives fulfilled." The reply included the following information.

The first year teaches the essentials of Christian discipleship, with the second year developing the teaching on ministry and leadership. Much of the focus on training for ministry is on developing a relationship with God and learning to be led by the Holy Spirit through the Word of God. People are trained to use the Bible as their "primary" resource, both in their own lives, and the lives of those they minister and care for.

The respondent named two books as being "some other resources that are used by the teaching staff in the general subject of pastoral care, incorporating the care of the mentally ill," as they "contain helpful principles that can be used in a variety of discipleship and pastoral situations."

With reference to the second investigative letter, the respondent from a Bible College replied that, "we do very little with regard to people with mental illness." He answered the questions quite specifically on training regarding general awareness of people with mental health problems and their care in that two or three hours of lectures were given in the care and counseling course, that there were occasionally guest speakers in chapel "on the subject," and that some students had visited Rampton hospital. He was not aware of any books or other teaching aids to help candidates familiarize themselves with the nature of mental illness. With reference to the questions on the Christian perspective, he stated that, "effectively we do nothing in these areas."

The second reply was from a Theological College. Students received lectures and guided reading concerning mental health problems, but did not visit hospitals. With regard to the distinctive Christian dimension, the College believed in "the personal, powerful and gracious support of God in Christ" and would therefore pray and encourage prayer. They brought a Christian awareness of the human spirit and the spiritual realm recognizing "the nature of spiritual blessing on the one hand and spiritual damage and attack on the other." The activities ordinarily expected of leaders in the course of their ministry would include prayer, visiting, pastoral counseling, and also the "general education of sufferers and carers about God and His ways towards fallen humanity." The training that the course provided was to assist people embarking on this work and included teaching about some selected common forms of mental illness and distress, and also practical training in basic counseling skills. It also included role-play and its assessment.

Conclusion

Although this study was based on a small sample because there are limited numbers of training colleges particularly of the Roman Catholic and Evangelical/Pentecostal denominations, it has been possible to show that there is an overall Christian attitude across all denominations in support of people with all kinds of sickness.

All denominations were, to some degree, involved in raising awareness of mental illness during the course of training at colleges. Literature, which included reference to mental illness, was available. Some Anglicans and Roman Catholics had access to clinical pastoral education. However, according to some of the leaders of the Evangelical/Pentecostal fellowships, the training in this area of pastoral care appeared to be sparse as they had little recollection of it and placed their reliance more on the Spirit and Christian instruction from the Bible.

It was difficult to assess the Christian perspective concerning mental illness because of lack of information particularly from the Anglican Church being unable to be specific due to pressure of time in responding. The Roman Catholics centered more on the dignity of the person, with Christ as a compassionate, sensitive, and listening, role model, and for students to be aware of Christ's outreach to the marginalized, and the essential inclusiveness of the Gospel. The Evangelical/Pentecostal colleges did not have a Christian perspective to their training with reference to people with mental illnesses, but believed in the power and support of God in Christ, and prayer.

I do believe that more needs to be done in the training of ministers in this area of pastoral ministry, specifically in view of the comments by the respondent of one of the Roman Catholic colleges and by leaders of the Evangelical/Pentecostal fellowships.

I now move forward by reporting the methodology used to obtain data on attitudes towards people with mental illnesses from Christian congregations of the same three ecclesial traditions.

Chapter 7

Methodology of research of attitudes in Christian congregations

All fieldwork research needs a method by which to collect its information, as well as a sample of people to approach in order to carry out the survey.

Survey method

My choice of instrument for my survey was the self-completion structured questionnaire. The advantages of this approach are that it is relatively cheap and requires very little time to administer. It allows anonymity in the responses as well as assuring reduction of interview bias, although no research method is without bias. A self-completion structured questionnaire is non-threatening as it can be completed in the privacy of one's home, and subjects can abstain without having to confront the researcher with their refusal. Large samples of people can be included, thus giving sufficient numbers of respondents to be "broad based" allowing the sample to be representative. It is an approach, tried and tested, and widely used for surveys.

A disadvantage of using a self-completion structured questionnaire is that the pre-coded response choices may not be sufficiently comprehensive and therefore respondents may choose inappropriate answers (Bowling, 1997). The data is more unreliable than face-to-face interviews as the researcher is not present to clarify points. Assumptions are made that the recipients can read and write, and questionnaires returned may be incorrectly filled in or incomplete. The notoriously low return from postal questionnaire surveys necessitates distribution of a large number of questionnaires in order to have enough returns to make the research viable (Edwards and Talbot, 1994).

There were other possible methods of research. For example, the approach where interviews take place, either by visiting on a one-to-one or telephoning, or in cluster groups, allow for more in-depth researching. However, the transcribing of all interviews, whether recorded or by tape or hand-written, is time consuming, and the analysis of the interviews is more difficult with in-depth research. While these different approaches were possibilities for my purpose, my choice of survey to collect information, after examining the advantages and disadvantages of each method, was the self-completed structured questionnaire, as it seemed the most suitable and practical. I had also used a similar method of investigation when exploring support for carers of people with mental illnesses as part of my research for my Masters degree, so was familiar with the method. As that particular piece of research contributed to a distinction for my dissertation, it seemed sensible to use a method, which had helped to produce a highly satisfactory piece of research.

Formation of questionnaire and letters

Careful thought, planning, and consultation, are very important for the design of a questionnaire before embarking on any fieldwork (Wilcox, 1998).

I initially drew on ideas for the design of the questionnaire from the model designed for my Masters. In formulating the first draft, I expanded these ideas. The literature survey spotlighted existing questionnaires and, in designing the questionnaire, I decided to use twenty-six statements on attitudes in relation to people with mental illnesses, from previous national surveys, to form section one of the questionnaire. These were extracted from an RSGB Omnibus survey prepared for the Department of Health (Department of Health, 1997). The advantage of using an existing questionnaire is that comparative data is available and, in this instance, would allow me to compare attitudes of the general public with those of Christian congregations. It would not be possible to make a true comparison between the data received from the two surveys because to do so would have meant targeting the same cross section of society for each survey. However, it would be possible to make some level of comparison between attitudes of Christian congregations with those of the general public.

Originally, the only intention was to explore perceptions, attitudes and understanding towards people with mental illnesses in Christian congregations. The questionnaire developed and expanded to include further sections on whether some beliefs provoked the causes of mental illnesses, and whether Christians considered themselves more prone to mental illnesses because of their religious beliefs. It also included sections on priority members of Christian congregations might give to address issues of mental illnesses within their congregations and in society in general, and possible ways of improving the integration of people with mental illnesses into faith communities. Prior to the main part of the questionnaire, there was a preliminary section to determine how informed Christians are at categorising illnesses in order to ascertain how knowledgeable they are in recognising what is a classed as a mental illness.

The wording, form and order of a questionnaire can all affect the type of responses obtained, and the skill of questionnaire design is to minimise influences and subsequent biases in the results (Bowling, 1997). The process of designing the questionnaire was rigorously carried out. I accessed wide-ranging methodological, medical, and theological resources, and included extensive piloting which is very important for directing possible changes necessary to instructions, question content, wording or sequence (Edwards and Talbot, 1994). This resulted in many modifications in format, wording, and content of the questionnaire, before arriving at the final copy.

I formulated a covering letter, to be sent to each of the distributors, explaining the nature of the study, reasons for the research, and outlining the procedure for the distribution and return of the questionnaires. I likewise drafted a courtesy letter, explaining the nature and scope of the study, to be sent to each of the four bishops, respectively, of the geographical region to be targeted. Again, consultation with the appropriate authorities led to modifications in format, wording, and content of the draft letters.

The sample and distribution

My decision was to limit the sample target to the three different ecclesial traditions referred to in the previous chapter, those of the Anglican Church, the Roman Catholic Church, and the Pentecostal/Evangelical fellowships, for reasons already given.

The area targeted was across two Anglican and two Roman Catholic dioceses of the northeast of England within which all three denominations were targeted. Respondents were identified through a variety of sources. For example, senior clergy of both the Anglican and Roman Catholic Churches were identified who had a wide knowledge of congregations throughout the targeted area as a result of their training responsibilities. They offered to help by supplying a list of parishes that were likely to support the study, and they further assisted by naming each priest in charge. Some Pentecostal and Evangelical fellowships were identified through the yellow pages directory, while others were suggested by these initial contacts. This is known as the snowballing technique, and is used where no sampling frame exists (Bowling, 1997).

Care was taken to ensure that the distribution of the questionnaires was across different parts of the chosen region covering rural and urban areas, coastal and countryside localities, and small and large congregations, by a selective choice of suggested distributors, in order to obtain as varied a sample as possible.

A set of questionnaires with a covering letter was sent to the leader of each congregation, either a priest or lay minister. Prior to the distribution, a copy of the letter for each of the bishops had been sent out. For both the Anglican and Roman Catholic denominations, a standard quota of questionnaires was sent to each parish, except where advice indicated that smaller or larger numbers would be appropriate. In the case of the Evangelical and Pentecostal fellowships, numbers were determined by telephoning each pastor or leader for advice. Fifteen hundred questionnaires were dispatched, but postal questionnaire surveys are notorious for their low response rate (Edwards and Talbot, 1994), and this proved to be the case in this instance.

Meanwhile, I was aware that I needed the necessary skills to transpose correctly the data from questionnaires to computer, and to be able to select and apply statistical techniques in order to analyse it. To this end, I enrolled on a Research Methods Course, which was available at the University of Teesside using the Statistical Package for Social Sciences (SPSS). SPSS is a package for the statistical analysis of data that is widely used in research, teaching and business (University of Durham, 1999). I attended weekly for the length of the course (one term).

Return

Five hundred and ninety-two questionnaires were returned, representing almost forty percent of the total distributed, satisfactory for a self-completion postal questionnaire survey.

I acknowledge that data collated from the questionnaires will not be truly representative of all United Kingdom Christian congregations as the questionnaires were distributed in a specific area. Data gathered from a certain area is not necessarily applicable to the whole. There was no specific instruction as to how the distributors should hand out the questionnaires. This meant possible bias towards regular committed attendees of places of worship or towards members of a specific setting such as a prayer group. However, I do not think that this is detrimental to gaining insights into attitudes towards people with mental illnesses in Christian congregations. It could be central to it because regular attendees are likely to be more aware than irregular ones of attitudes within their congregations.

Having detailed the method of research and the sample, I continue my study by presenting in the next chapter a comparison of attitudes of members of Christian congregations towards people with mental illnesses with those of the general public. Will I find that being a Christian makes a difference?

Chapter 8

Comparison of attitudes of Christians with those of the general public towards people with mental illnesses

This chapter presents the outcome of the investigation into attitudes of Christians towards people with mental illnesses by comparing them with those of the general public.

Categorizing illnesses

Prior to reporting on the investigation, I wanted to look at how informed the Christian respondents are at designating illnesses to named categories. The reason for this was to ascertain how knowledgeable the respondents are in recognizing what is classed as a mental illness. This will establish whether or not there is a consensus of agreement between the respondents on categorizing illnesses. If there is a high consensus of agreement, this will add strength to the results of the questionnaire, because the respondents will have been thinking along similar lines when formulating their responses.

The method used to carry out this investigation was to utilize part of the self-completion questionnaire referred to in the chapter on methodology. Prior to the main part of the questionnaire, the respondents were presented with a list of eighteen illnesses associated with mental illnesses and learning disabilities. The respondents were invited to indicate, by ticking the appropriate box, which of the three categories of "mental illness," "mental handicap," or "other," they believed the illness belonged. Hopefully, this would help them establish and internalize their personal understanding of a mental illness before responding to the questionnaire proper. The illnesses were placed in alphabetical order in the questionnaire to help counteract bias. To test the accuracy of the results, the responses were compared with the classification of illnesses by the worldwide authority, the World Health Organization (1992).

Results

The percentages of respondents indicating an illness to be a mental illness, and also whether or not the illness is a mental illness according to the World Health Organization (WHO), are displayed below.

Illness	Mental illness	WHO	Illness	Mental illness	WHO
Schizophrenia	93.40%	yes	Epilepsy	13.30%	no
Manic depression	86.40%	yes	Parkinson's	11.30%	no
Clinical depression	82.80%	yes	Motor neurone	9.70%	no
Obsessive-compulsive	77.20%	yes	Cerebal palsy	7.40%	no
Anorexia/bulimia	67.70%	yes	Downs syndrome	5.00%	no
Alzheimer's disease	65.70%	yes	Cystic fibrosis	3.50%	no
Post-traumatic stress	63.10%	yes	Multiple sclerosis	3.10%	no
Anxiety	52.60%	yes	Diabetes	2.40%	no
Autism	18.90%	yes	Muscular dystrophy	1.80%	no

A very high percentage of respondents indicated that schizophrenia was a mental illness, and more than eighty percent indicated the same for manic depression and clinical depression. Over seventy-five percent of respondents signified that obsessive-compulsive disorder was a mental illness with slightly lesser percentages signifying this of anorexia/bulimia, Alzheimer's disease and post-traumatic stress disorder. Finally, a little more than fifty percent of the respondents indicated that anxiety was a mental illness. However, just less than twenty percent of respondents thought that autism was a mental illness.

According to the leading authority on classification of mental disorders, eight of the illnesses indicated to be mental illnesses by more than half of the respondents and a much higher percentage in most instances, are mental disorders. With reference to Alzheimer's disease, note that the American Psychiatric Association (1994), in DSM-IV on mental disorders, makes reference to a dementia of the Alzheimer's type in its section on dementia.

The results show that an absolute minimal percentage of respondents considered muscular dystrophy, diabetes, multiple sclerosis and cystic fibrosis to be mental illnesses. A very small percentage indicated this of Downs syndrome and cerebral palsy, and percentages increased only slightly with regard to motor neurone disease, Parkinson's disease and epilepsy.

The World Health Organization (1992) makes reference to multiple sclerosis, Downs syndrome, Parkinson's disease and epilepsy. It does not classify them as mental illnesses but lists them under other conditions often associated with mental and behavioral disorders. This leaves muscular dystrophy, diabetes, cystic fibrosis, cerebral palsy and motor neurone disease not mentioned by WHO in this particular classification of illnesses. The absence of these illnesses in the clinical description and diagnostic guidelines of the ICD-10 Classification of Mental and Behavioral Disorders shows that the respondents were correct in their assumptions that these illnesses were not mental illnesses. This authority is an exhaustive classification with very widespread professional acceptance based on evidence on the same lines, and it would have classified them had they been mental illnesses.

A high ratio of respondents, in their indications of whether or not seventeen of the eighteen illnesses listed were mental illnesses, was correct according to the World Health Organization. This indicates that generally the respondents were well informed. Regarding the remaining one, slightly more than four-fifths of the respondents were in agreement that the illness was not a mental illness (although in fact it is). In other words, the results showed that there was a high degree of consensus of opinion amongst the respondents overall in their understanding of what they believe to be a mental illness.

Age

The next step was to investigate whether age was a determining variable in any differences of opinion on categorizing the illnesses.

The respondents, when presented with the questionnaire, were invited as a preliminary to the questionnaire proper, to indicate in which of four age brackets they belonged. The age brackets and the percentages of each age group are displayed below.

Age bracket
18-30: 6.30%   31-50: 37.60%   51-70: 42.00%
71plus: 14.10%

Almost eighty percent of all respondents were of the middle two age groups. Of the remainder, more than twice as many respondents were in the oldest age group compared with those of the youngest age group.

The average of totals of percentages of each age bracket was calculated, and results are displayed below.

Average of responses within age groups
18-30   31-50   51-70   71plus

9 illnesses indicated as mental illnesses
67.42%   70.78%   68.60%   58.95%

9 illnesses not indicated as mental illnesses
12.83%   6.24%   5.40%   6.92%

Respondents of age groups 31-50 and 51-70 were in close agreement in what they considered to be mental illnesses. There was similar agreement between respondents of these same age groups on illnesses not considered to be mental illnesses. The respondents aged 18-30 agreed in the first instance with those of the 31-50 and 51-70 age groups, unlike those aged 71plus. In the second instance, it was the respondents aged 71plus that concurred with those of the 31-50 and 51-70 age groups, unlike those aged 18-30.

Given that almost eighty percent of all respondents were in the two middle age groups, this meant that four of every five had a similar understanding of what is classed as a mental illness. Generally, the respondents were well informed, and there was a high degree of consensus of opinion.

Comparison of attitudes of Christians with those of the general public

Having established that overall, the respondents were well informed about indicating what was a mental illness, and that the tests by age confirmed that a large majority was of a similar mind, I continue by comparing attitudes of members of Christian congregations with those of the general public towards people with mental illnesses.

In order to make this comparison, participants were asked to respond to a set twenty-six questions that have been used in regular surveys on behalf of the Department of Health since 1993. The respondents of the Christian congregations were drawn from three ecclesial traditions as catalogued in the previous chapter. They were volunteers. The comparison group of the RSGB General Omnibus Survey, on behalf of the Department of Health, comprised a national representative sample of two thousand adults surveyed in 2000, and the relevant data was accessed from the RSGB report (Department of Health, 2000) for the purpose of this report.

The twenty-six statements covered a range of issues on attitudes towards people with mental illnesses to opinions on services provided for people with the illnesses. The wording of three statements was altered to remove gender specificity, the words "woman" or "man" being replaced by "person" or "someone." Other thirteen statements had minimal alterations. These changes were done on the basis of ethical advice. In other respects, the statements were identical. The twenty-six statements were placed in the same mixed up order in the survey as those of the RSGB General Omnibus Survey.

Christian respondents were asked to rate each statement on a five-point attitude scale, while respondents of the survey on behalf of Department of Health were given a six-point response scale, as displayed below. Throughout this report, CC denotes the Christian respondents and DH those of the general public.

CC agree strongly	agree slightly	neither agree/disagree	disagree slightly	disagree strongly	
DH agree strongly	agree slightly	neither agree/disagree	disagree slightly	disagree strongly	don't know

For the purposes of analysis, each statement was allocated to one of four classifications. I had based three of the classifications on examples by Wolff *et al* (1996c) and the other from examples by Corrigan *et al* (2001).

Classifications were labeled Fear and Exclusion, Familiarity, Social Control, and Goodwill. Each statement was inspected and an attempt was made to identify underlying themes in order to place each statement within one of the classifications.

Firstly, percentages of majority responses to each of the twenty-six components of both surveys were compared statistically. Secondly, responses to each of the twenty-six components within each survey were allocated to either neutral, agree, or disagree, as displayed below, collated and compared. This was to determine how much neutrality there was in responding, and to see if this was linked with differences of opinion where definite responses had been given.

CC	neutral	=	neither agree/disagree
DH	neutral	=	neither agree/disagree/don't know
CC and DH	agree	=	agree strongly/agree slightly
CC and DH	disagree	=	disagree slightly/disagree strongly

Fear and Exclusion was the first classification examined in this section

Fear and Exclusion
Less emphasis should be placed on protecting the public from people with mental illnesses
No one has the right to exclude people with mental illnesses from their neighborhood
People with mental illnesses are far less of a danger than most people suppose
As far as possible, mental health services should be provided through community based facilities
The best therapy for many people with mental illnesses is to be part of a "normal" community
Residents have nothing to fear from people coming into their neighborhood to obtain mental health services
It is frightening to think of people with mental illnesses living in residential neighborhoods

Locating mental health facilities in a residential area downgrades the neighborhood

The results of the statistical tests of the Fear and Exclusion classification showed that significant differences arose between the Christian respondents and those of the general public on responses to three of these components. The three components in question are displayed below.

The best therapy for many people with mental illnesses is to be part of a "normal" community
Residents have nothing to fear from people coming into their neighborhood to obtain mental health services
It is frightening to think of people with mental illnesses living in residential neighborhoods

It is apparent that these differences arose on issues of specified fear of proximity of people with mental illnesses. On each of the differences arising, the Christian respondents had a higher percentage of more favorable responses towards people with mental illnesses than those of the general public. There were no significant differences arising on the remaining components but the contact implied was not quite as specific.

The results suggest that the Christian respondents were of a similar mind to those of the general public in responding to the more general components, but were more accepting of the proximity of people with mental illnesses as demonstrated in the statistical differences.

There was a high level of uncertainty in responses to some components. For example, on the following component displayed, well over twenty-five percent of respondents were unable to be definite, with over a thirty-four percent agreeing and, likewise, disagreeing.

Less emphasis should be placed on protecting the public from people with mental illnesses
neutral   CC 28.53% DH 30.41%   agree CC 36.25% DH 34.09%
disagree   CC 35.22% DH 35.50%

This shows that large percentages of respondents were unsure of how to respond, and the remaining respondents were almost equally divided into for or against, demonstrating how diverse were the opinions of all respondents over the element of danger when encountering people with mental illnesses.

There was a high percentage of approximately twenty percent of Christian respondents unsure on how to respond to a further three components by neither agreeing nor disagreeing, and similarly with those of the general public but on a further five components. Only on one component of the eight, were there slightly less than ten percent of the Christian respondents indecisive in responding but, even then, it was over ten percent of the respondents of the general public who were uncertain. On all but one component, the Christian respondents were slightly less indecisive in their responses than those of the general public.

Prejudicial and NIMBY attitudes towards people with mental illnesses alongside stigmatization, surfaced from the survey of literature and results of research reported in earlier chapters. The survey also revealed discrimination in all walks of life and general social exclusion and isolation. These attitudes were perceived by members of the general public and confirmed by the users of mental health services. The survey also exposed fear, lack of knowledge, and unfamiliarity with people with mental illnesses, all of which contributed to unfavorable attitudes that were possibly increased by negative output of the media and attitudes of the medical profession.

The results of this current survey have confirmed that there is still much fear with regard to mental illness.

This was my own experience when I worked at the mental health day center in the 1990s. For example, in a conversation on the telephone with my sister-in-law, I told her where I was working and that people at the center included those with schizophrenia. Her reaction was to question whether I was frightened that they might do something.

Koenig (2005) illustrates a situation in Minnesota where the first question asked of a mother of her son, diagnosed with schizophrenia and who has requested a visit from a priest, was to enquire if he was violent. Koenig states that fear, ignorance and shame often prevent people from talking about mental illness even though, he adds, mental illnesses affect one in four Minnesota families.

Familiarity was the next classification examined in this section

Familiarity
A person would be foolish to marry someone who has had a mental illness even though he/she seems fully recovered
I would not want to live next door to someone who has been mentally ill
Most people who have been patients in mental hospitals can be trusted as baby-sitters

The results of the statistical tests showed that significant differences arose between the Christian respondents and those of the general public on responses to all components of the Familiarity classification. A closer examination of the content showed that the differences arose on specific personal contact with people with mental illnesses. In each case, there were more Christian respondents open to personal contact with people with mental illnesses and with accepting attitudes towards them than those of the general public. These results reinforce the outcome of responses within the classification of Fear and Exclusion.

Where there was great uncertainty, there was diversity of opinions on agreeing or disagreeing, for example, to the component displayed below.

Most people who have been patients in mental hospitals can be trusted as baby-sitters
neutral   CC 35.96% DH 38.44%   agree CC 27.74% DH 19.35%
disagree CC 36.30% DH 42.21%

In response to this component, more than a thirty-five percent of the respondents were unable to be definite, and there were major conflicts of opinion between respondents in agreeing or in disagreeing. This component gave rise to the highest percentages, from results to all components, of those unable to be definite in their responses.

Of the other two components, there were almost a twenty-five percent of Christian respondents who were either uncertain, or disagreed with the first component, and almost twenty percent with reference to the second component. Percentages increased with reference to the respondents of the general public. Approximately thirty-three percent were unsure or disagreed with the first component and well more than a twenty-five percent likewise of the second component. The Christian respondents were less uncertain in their responses to all components in this classification than those of the general public.

Edna Hunneysett

The issue of babysitting, when our teenage daughter, Elizabeth, was seriously ill with severe clinical depression, is revealed in my story.

"Hello, Edna, it's Katie." She always sounded so cheerful on the telephone. "Edna, I wondered how Elizabeth is? I was going to have a word with her? Is she able to baby-sit?" Katie was a friend of many years standing. She had two children and when needing a babysitter would call on Elizabeth. Katie's daughter, Mary, now eleven, would have no other person to sit when her parents were out. She was delighted when Elizabeth went to their home. Katie admitted to not understanding Elizabeth's illness, but when needing a baby-sitter, rang and spoke to either myself, or Elizabeth. Katie trusted my judgment implicitly as to whether or not Elizabeth was well enough. I would either pass the telephone to Elizabeth, or if she was ill I would ask her and she would tell me herself if she felt unable to baby-sit. There were times when I knew it was unnecessary to discuss it with her; she was just too ill. This was one of them.

"I'm sorry Katie; she is not well enough. She is quite poorly at present." Katie accepted the situation graciously and sympathetically.

It was great affirmation for Elizabeth that Katie and her husband, Patrick, totally accepted and trusted Elizabeth and treated her like any normal person who occasionally was too ill to be of help. Katie told me of an incident when comments had came back to her about Elizabeth and how she had tried to rectify damage that might be caused to Elizabeth. She wanted me to hear so as to make sure she was explaining the facts correctly. Apparently, on one of the occasions when it had been arranged for Elizabeth to baby-sit, Katie's thirteen year old son, John, had been asked by a friend at school the name of their baby-sitter. When John told him, his friend questioned him.

"Elizabeth Hunneysett?"

"Yes," John replied.

"Well," retorted his friend, "she should not be baby-sitting; she has had a breakdown." John reported this conversation to his mother and she had sat him down and explained the nature of Elizabeth's illness as best she could.

"Is that what it is?" John replied. "Then she's okay to sit, isn't she?"

"Yes, and when you next see your friend, you tell him the facts," his mother added. What Katie had helped him to realize was that Elizabeth was quite able to baby-sit when well; that there was nothing sinister about her illness (Hunneysett, 2009).

Social Control was the next classification examined in this section

Social Control
One of the main causes of a mental illness is lack of self-discipline and willpower
There is something about people with mental illnesses that makes it easy to tell them from "normal" people
As soon as a person shows signs of mental disturbance he/she should be hospitalized
Mental hospitals are an outdated means of treating people with mental illnesses
Increased spending on mental health services is a waste of money
There are sufficient existing services for people with mental illnesses
People with mental illnesses should not be given any responsibility
Anyone with a history of mental problems should be excluded from taking public office

The results of the statistical tests showed that significant differences arose between the Christian respondents and those of the general public on responses to six components of the Social Control classification. In all instances of significant differences, the Christian respondents showed a more liberal attitude than those of the general public, suggesting that they were more inclined to acceptance of the equality of people with mental illnesses. There were underlying issues that were subjective. In some cases, the content of components was more authoritarian in attitude showing the Christian respondents to be less authoritarian than those of the general public. Some examples of results are given below.

People with mental illnesses should not be given any responsibility
neutral   CC 15.04% DH 23.34%   agree CC 8.89% DH 13.67%
disagree CC 76.07% DH 62.99%

Anyone with a history of mental problems should be excluded from taking public office
neutral   CC 20.35% DH 23.95%   agree CC 17.26% DH 24.26%
disagree CC 62.39% DH 51.79%

Of the two components of the Social Control classification that gave rise to no significant differences, the content was of a more general nature relevant to people with mental illness. However, there was evidence of uncertainty in giving definite responses, as displayed in an example below, where more than twenty-one percent of Christian respondents, and almost twenty-five percent of those of the general public, were uncertain about the issue.

Mental hospitals are an outdated means of treating people with mental illnesses

neutral CC 21.92% DH 24.96%   agree CC 41.44% DH 40.29%
disagree CC 36.64% DH 34.75%

The greatest difference in uncertainty between respondents of the two surveys, was on the results of the component displayed below, demonstrating a much more informed attitude by the Christian respondents.

One of the main causes of a mental illness is lack of self-discipline and willpower
neutral   CC   7.00% DH 20.33%   agree CC 6.65% DH 13.26%
disagree CC 86.35% DH 66.41%

The Christian respondents were less indecisive in responses to all components of the Social Control classification than those of the general public.

The research detailed in earlier chapters revealed discrimination of people with mental illnesses in all aspects of life.
According to Address (2003), there are great inequities in the United States between coverage of mental health care and physical health care.

Goodwill was the final classification examined in this section

Goodwill
Mental illness is an illness like any other
Virtually anyone can become mentally ill
People with mental illnesses have for too long been the subject of ridicule
There is need to adopt a far more tolerant attitude towards people with mental illnesses in our communities
We have a responsibility to provide the best possible care for people with mental illnesses. People with mental illnesses don't deserve our sympathy
People with mental illnesses are a burden on society

The results of the statistical tests showed that significant differences arose between the Christian respondents and those of the general public on responses from the results of three of the components of the Goodwill classification where more tolerance and a responsibility to provide the best possible care were the key issues. An example is given below.

People with mental illnesses don't deserve our sympathy
neutral CC 1.70% DH 5.75%   agree CC 2.22% DH 5.09%
disagree CC 96.08% DH 89.16%

Where differences arose, it was the Christian respondents who were more caring and accepting in attitude in their responses than those of the general public.

There were no significant differences on results to four components, the issues of which were of a more general nature relevant to people with mental illnesses, as, for example, in the results to one component displayed below.

Virtually anyone can become mentally ill
neutral CC 2.38% DH 5.05%   agree CC 94.21% DH 92.33%
disagree CC 3.41% DH 2.62%

Generally, there were very high percentages of both the Christian respondents and those of the general public, in results to four components, who were benevolently disposed towards people with mental illnesses and of the remaining three, high percentages demonstrated favorable responses. Nevertheless, on a sliding scale, there was twenty to ten percent of Christian respondents and slightly more of those of the general public who were uncertain in attitude, or not as benevolent.

There was little indecisiveness in responding to these components possibly because the components were more general in their content, and general components require less understanding and allow for more positive responses, thus allowing for less soul searching decisions.

Overall, from the results of statistical tests, the differences between the respondents of the two surveys were not significant on eleven of the twenty-six components, but there were significant and very significant differences on the remaining fifteen components.

I need to consider now whether these differences are because of Christian influence or whether there were other underlying factors that may have played a part where Christian respondents were more positive and accepting that those of the general public towards people with mental illnesses. My investigation continues.

Age

The sub group age was the first to be investigated to determine if it was an underlying factor that may have played a part in the differences detailed earlier between the surveys.

Percentages of respondents of each age group of each survey were collated for comparison. It was evident from the results that there was a greater percentage of older respondents of the Christian congregations survey than those of the national survey.

Percentages of supportive responses to the components of each of the classifications detailed earlier, were collated and tested statistically by age. The tests demonstrated that it was the respondents of the younger and older age groups of both surveys, but slightly more so the older age groups, that were less accepting in their attitude towards people with mental illnesses.

As the respondents of the Christian communities were of an older age than those of the survey on behalf of the Department of Health, and as the older age groups were shown to be less favorable in attitude, it would be expected that results overall would show Christian respondents to be less favorable in attitude than those of the general public but in fact the opposite was true. Therefore, age, as a subgroup, did not appear to estimate a likely direction of any bias reflected in the differences arising from the responses to the two surveys.

This similarly applies to the economic status because percentages of respondents of different economic categories revealed that there was a larger proportion of retired respondents within the Christian communities sample than of the survey on behalf of the Department of Health.

Gender

The sub group gender was the next to be investigated.

Percentages of female and male respondents of both surveys were collated. There were more females than males in both surveys. There was a greater percentage of female respondents in the Christian congregations survey than of the general public survey and, consequently, a lower percentage of corresponding males.

Percentages of favorable responses to the components of each of the classifications detailed earlier, were collated and tested statistically by gender. The results of the tests by gender gave rise to five significant differences within the Christians congregations survey and one of those was borderline, and to four within the survey on behalf of the Department of Health.

In conclusion, as differences by gender had not arisen from the majority of the twenty-six components, this implied that female and male respondents had similar attitudes. This suggested that it was not the fact of females or males having different attitudes that had given rise to the fifteen statistically significant differences between the results of the two surveys. Therefore, as females and males responded similarly in each survey, gender, as a subgroup, did not appear to be the underlying factor that estimated a likely direction of any bias reflected in the differences arising from the responses to the two surveys.

Geographical region

It may have been that living in the geographical region of the northeast of England, as in the case of the respondents of the Christian congregations, was an underlying factor that may have played a part in the differences detailed earlier between the surveys. This possibility was investigated.

It was noted that the Christian congregations were sampled within two of the regions covered by the nation survey. Thus, these two regions of the general public survey coincided with the geographical area of the sampling of the Christian congregations. This allowed for some comparison to determine whether living in the northeast introduced any bias within the differences that had arisen between the responses of the two surveys.

Consequently, as a measure for comparison, the results specifically of the region of the northeast of England of the survey on behalf of the Department of Health were compared with those of its entire national survey. This was to determine whether the respondents of the northeast region of the general public survey had similar attitudes as those countrywide. If they held similar attitudes, then living in the northeast of England would not be expected to introduce a likely direction of bias within the statistically significant differences arising from the results of the Christian survey and those of the survey on behalf of the Department of Health.

The outcome of the statistical tests showed little differences in opinion between the respondents of the northeast region of England of the national survey, and those of the whole national survey. Results within the four classifications showed statistically significant differences arising on results to only six components out of a possible twenty-six compared with fifteen of the components when comparing the Christian responses to those of the respondents of the entire survey on behalf of the Department of Health. The conclusion was that the estimated likely direction of any bias was not because the Christian respondents lived in the geographical region of the northeast of England

Carers/People having experienced mental illness

Another joint subgroup investigated was carers and sufferers, as carers of people with mental illnesses and those who themselves have experienced a mental illness may estimate a likely direction of bias.

Percentages of respondents of both surveys who had indicated that they were either carers of people with mental illnesses or who had themselves experienced a mental illness were collated, and percentages by gender were also collated, as displayed below.

Carers CC 26.90% DH: 24%   female CC 28.60%   DH 26.00%
                                                                            male   CC 23.40%   DH 22.00%
Experienced mental illness
          CC 14.90% DH 13%   female CC 16.00%   DH 16.00%

male   CC 12.60%   DH 10.00%

It is evident that percentages from both surveys were very similar. Therefore, these two groups would not appear to be the factor in my survey influencing the more favorable attitudes.

Conclusion

The differences on comparison of results tested statistically showed that the respondents of the Christian congregations had a more accepting and supportive attitude towards people with mental illnesses than those of the national survey in each situation where differences had arisen. Sub groups of respondents were investigated where possible to estimate the likely direction of any bias in these differences. No evidence of an estimated likely direction of any bias within the statistically differences arising between the results of the two surveys by age, gender and geographical region, had been identified.

The differences had arisen on issues, concerning people with mental illnesses, of fear of proximity; of specific personal contact; of consideration of equality; and of explicit positive attitudes, rather than general issues related to mental illness. The profiles of the Christian respondents showed that a very high percentage attended a place of worship weekly or more often. Thus, almost all the respondents of the Christian congregations were regularly listening to biblical teaching on the foundational concept of loving one's neighbor as oneself as well, as well as participating in worship and prayer. It is therefore, reasonable to suggest that Christianity played a major part in the more accepting attitudes shown by the Christian respondents when compared with the attitudes of the general public.

These results are similar to those of a much smaller survey, detailed in an earlier chapter, undertaken to measure attitudes of members of a congregation at a standard Sunday church service of a predominantly white, middle class, evangelical Anglican community (Gray, 2001). They are also consistent with Gill's discovery that churchgoers are significantly different from non-churchgoers. Gill argues that churchgoers have higher levels of Christian belief but, in addition, they "usually have a stronger sense of moral and civic order and tend to be significantly more altruistic than non-churchgoers" (Gill, 1999: 261).

Friedli (2000) believes that religious communities are often in the front line with regard to care and means of support, and that for those isolated or unsupported, their place of worship, be it the church, mosque, or synagogue, may be the only place where they can meet socially, and one of the few sources of information and support. There is, she points out, a need to investigate the extent of which people with mental illnesses are silenced or excluded from their faith communities, and the parallel failure of mental health services to acknowledge and respect people's religious and spiritual needs. Friedli suggests that a shift from the emphasis of faith communities being providers of support to being mental health promoters has great potential, and because of the experiences of many within faith communities who have experienced mental health problems, she believes that faith communities have an important role in increasing understanding of mental health issues and challenging stigma and discrimination.

In conclusion, from the results of responses to the twenty-six components, the Christian respondents were more tolerant and accepting in attitude than those, overall, of the general public where there were significant differences. However, the results do not mean that the majority of Christian respondents had positive attitudes in all instances. The Christian respondents had less responses of neutrality than those of the general public and alongside this, less divergence of responses, but still sufficient to reveal dilemmas and division of opinion. This confirms that respondents did not know how to respond to some components and this indecisiveness implies lack of knowledge or understanding. The results suggest that had the respondents been better informed about issues surrounding mental illness, there would have been fewer indecisive responses and more consensus of opinion. This points to a need for education in raising awareness and understanding.

This concludes the comparison between attitudes of the general public with those of the Christian respondents. I now move forward to investigate and compare attitudes towards members with mental illnesses of respondents of Christian congregations of three different ecclesial traditions, and I present the results in the next chapter. Does belonging to a different denomination make a difference in attitude?

Chapter 9

Research of Christian attitudes today towards people with mental illnesses

In this chapter, I investigate attitudes of Christians towards people with mental illnesses in their congregations and compare the attitudes of members from three ecclesial traditions. I also compare attitudes and spiritual beliefs, and attitudes on possible proneness to mental illnesses because of Christian faith.

Attitudes within Christian congregations

My first enquiry concerns attitudes within Christian congregations towards members with mental illnesses.

The approach used was the same self-completion questionnaire and respondents were presented with a sheet within the questionnaire containing a set of fourteen statements listed in random order. These covered a range of issues on attitudes towards, and support offered, to people with mental illnesses in Christian congregations. The respondents were asked to rate each statement on the five-point attitude scale, described and displayed in the previous chapter.

For the purposes of analysis, each statement was allocated to one of three classifications of Stigma, Social Control, and Goodwill. Each statement was inspected and an attempt was made to identify underlying themes in order to place each statement within one of the classifications.

Following this, percentages of favorable responses to each of the fourteen components were compared statistically. Secondly, responses to each of the fourteen components were allocated to either neutral, agree, or disagree as displayed in the previous chapter, collated and compared. This was to determine how much neutrality there was in responding, and whether this was linked with differences of opinion where definite responses were given.

Stigma was the first classification examined in this section

Stigma
People with mental illnesses including those in Christian communities have to deal with not only the illness but also the associated stigma
Relatives caring for persons with mental illnesses in Christian communities have to cope with the associated stigma of having a relative with a mental illness

There was a very significant difference between the denominations on responses to one component of the classification of Stigma, as shown below.

Relatives caring for persons with mental illnesses in Christian communities have to cope with the associated stigma of having a relative with a mental illness

Anglican 57.10% Roman Catholic 60.40%
Evangelical/Pentecostal 42.80%

Only slightly more than forty-two percent of the Evangelical/Pentecostal respondents agreed to this component, whereas approximately fifty-seven percent of the Anglicans and a slightly higher percentage of Roman Catholics agreed.

The responses to this same component also showed that almost twenty percent of all respondents were unable to give a definite opinion, leaving approximately twenty-five percent of respondents disagreeing. Of the other component of the Stigma classification, there was a high consensus of just over eighty percent of respondents in agreement with it. Just over ten percent of respondents were unable to be definite in their responses to this component, and it was less than ten percent who disagreed with it. Thus, the results demonstrate that many of the respondents believe that stigma is prevalent in their Christian congregations.

The literature survey and results of research reported in earlier chapters also revealed that stigma has detrimental consequences on the lives of people with mental illnesses including negative effects on families, carers and relatives.

Koenig (2005) reports that in America, there is a barrier of stigma especially among the elderly because of how others might perceive them. For younger patients, they are concerned about future job opportunities since many applications require that a person mention whether or not he or she has ever needed mental health care, and there is also concern as to how friends at church will view them. (Address, 2003) agrees that the reality is that mental illness continues to be stigmatized in their society, and people with mental illness are frequently the objects of ridicule, contempt, or fear, and are frequently marginalized and excluded.

Social Control was the next classification examined in this section

Social Control
Most members in Christian communities give people with mental illnesses priority when supporting people in need
People with mental illnesses and their families in Christian communities are given care equal to that given to the other sick people and their families

Pastoral Care: Mental Health

Most Christian communities give priority in terms of resources to people with mental illnesses

There are adequate existing supports for people with mental illnesses in most Christian communities

Christian communities have an obligation to help support people with mental illnesses and their families

Christian communities need to allocate resources to helping people with mental illnesses

Very significant differences arose between the denominations of the favorable results to three of the six components of the classification of Social Control, as displayed below.

Christian communities have an obligation to help support people with mental illnesses and their families
Anglican   86.90%   Roman Catholic   89.20%
Evangelical/Pentecostal   76.60%

Christian communities need to allocate resources to helping people with mental illnesses
Anglican   75.20%   Roman Catholic   81.50%
Evangelical/Pentecostal   65.60%

People with mental illnesses and their families in Christian communities are given care equal to that given to the other sick people and their families
Anglican   41.10%   Roman Catholic   35.00%
Evangelical/Pentecostal   52.40%

There was evidence of uncertainty by respondents in giving definite responses to components of the classification of Social Control, as percentages of respondents indicate, shown in examples displayed below.

Most members in Christian communities give people with mental illnesses priority when supporting people in need
neutral 30.80%   agree 33.60%   disagree 35.60%

People with mental illnesses and their families in Christian communities are given care equal to that given to the other sick people and their families
neutral 23.50%   agree 41.30%   disagree 35.20%

There are adequate existing supports for people with mental illnesses in most Christian communities.
neutral 19.10%   agree 10.80%   disagree 70.10%

These results show that respondents are unsure about help on offer but, of the last of these components displayed above, it is evident that the respondents feel that whatever the support for people with mental illnesses they are aware of, they believe it is insufficient.

Koenig reports from America, of a psychiatrist stating that church members are encouraged to keep mental health problems hidden and that mental illness is still a taboo subject in many places, that many faith-based groups "still don't recognize that providing social support and other mental health resources can really help prevent, hasten recovery from, or stabilize mental illness" (Koenig, 2005: 253).

Sutherland (1999) offers a framework within which the resources of the Christian tradition might be made available to those who suffer from mental health problems. He believes that outside of the criminal justice system, poor mental health is the major symbol of exclusion in society and argues for a dialogue between psychiatry and the religious tradition. He believes that there is an urgent need for the resources of the religious tradition to be both better understood, and made more widely available, to those who suffer with poor mental health.

Goodwill was the final classification examined in this section

Goodwill
People with mental illnesses in Christian communities are marginalized by most other members
The vast majority of members in Christian communities remain indifferent towards people with mental illnesses and their families
Members of Christian communities need to adopt a more embracing attitude towards people with mental illnesses
Most members of Christian communities fail to express Christ-like concern to people with mental illnesses
Most Christian communities allow people with mental illnesses to become invisible
Christ-like concern towards people with mental illnesses is evident in the majority of Christian communities today

Significant differences arose between the responses of the denominations to only one component of the classification of Goodwill, as displayed below.

Christ-like concern towards people with mental illnesses is evident in the majority of Christian communities today
Anglican 28.50% Roman Catholic 37.70%
Evangelical/Pentecostal 39.50%

Also, with regard to this component in agreeing, disagreeing and being uncertain, all the respondents were almost equally divided in their responses. Respondents had very diverse opinions, and much uncertainty in their responses to a further four components where approximately twenty-five percent of respondents were unable to give definite responses and there were large divisions of opinion by the remainder of respondents in agreeing or disagreeing. The one remaining component gave rise to a large majority of favorable responses, the results of which are displayed below.

Members of Christian communities need to adopt a more embracing attitude towards people with mental illnesses
neutral 12.00%　　agree 82.70%　　disagree 5.30%

Overall, in this section, the results showed that attitudes and understanding between Christian denominations were similar in a majority of examples with significant differences between the denominations on results from only five of the fourteen components. Of two of these, the majority percentages of respondents in agreement were already high but of the other three, the majority percentages involved were around fifty percent or less of the respondents. Where these five differences occurred, in each situation except one, the Anglican and Roman Catholic respondents were more in union with each other in agreeing or disagreeing than with the respondents of the Evangelical/Pentecostal fellowships. For example, a lesser percentage of the Evangelical/Pentecostal respondents thought that the relatives of those with mental illnesses had associated stigma to cope with than of the other two denominations, and a greater percentage thought that equal care was given than of the Anglican and Roman Catholic respondents. A lesser percentage thought that there was an obligation to support and of the need to allocate resources than of the Anglican and Roman Catholic respondents. Of the fifth component, it was a lesser percentage of the Anglican respondents who agreed that Christ-like concern was evident than of the other two denominations.

These results suggest that that the Evangelical/Pentecostal respondents disagreed less on more support needed because they felt that equal care was being given to all sick people including those with mental illnesses. It does appear that these results may imply a possible fundamental denominational difference concerning some issues relating to mental illness or that, because the fabrication of the Evangelical/Pentecostal fellowships is generally much smaller than those of the Anglicans and Roman Catholics, and with usually only one gathering for weekend services compared with more than one within Anglican and Roman Catholic communities, it is conceivable that people with mental illnesses are able to feel more visible and known in smaller fellowships, and consequently, possibly feel more accepted and supported.

Of the fourteen components, only five gave rise to majority percentages of approximately seventy to eighty-six percent of respondents who were in agreement on a given component. A good majority agreed that there was a stigma attached to having a mental illness. The majority of respondents disagreed that there were adequate supports, and agreed that there was an obligation to help and to allocate resources, and that there was need to adopt more embracing attitudes. All of these issues were of a general nature. This implied that attitudes and understanding were similar and favorable in Christian congregations where issues referred to were not explicit in definition.

The remaining nine components gave rise to much smaller majorities of less than thirty percent to slightly more than a fifty-five percent of the respondents agreeing or disagreeing, as greater percentages of respondents were unsure in their responses. There was uncertainty by almost twenty percent of the respondents about relatives being subjected to stigma. There were percentages of almost twenty-three to thirty-four percent of respondents uncertain with regard to priority of support, priority of resources, and equal care in relation to people with mental illnesses. These three components were specific in content about the precise nature and quality of the suggested support by the Christian congregations. Other components, that they were unsure about or disagreed over, were most explicit in citing the situation such as marginalization; indifference; failure to express Christ-like concern, and whether this concern was visible; and whether people with mental illnesses were allowed to become invisible. Thus, there were many instances where respondents were unsure or disagreed over the issues showing that there were uncertain and diverse opinions amongst the Christians.

The majority of the respondents seemed confident that people with mental illnesses should be supported but much less sure of whether this took place within their congregations. These results suggest that the respondents were unaware of the situation on many issues relating to people with mental illnesses in Christian congregations. It has already been demonstrated that the majority of respondents were in agreement over what constituted a mental illness. In order to make an informed response to the classifications of Stigma, Social Control and Goodwill, being acquainted with people with mental illnesses in the Christian congregations would be a necessary contributory factor in determining a definite response. This raises the question of how hidden are mental illnesses in Christian congregations.

Results of research carried out in the UK, USA and Alaska, reported in earlier chapters, revealed the importance of religious and spiritual beliefs in providing meaning in various ways for people with mental illnesses. For a few, their religious faith was one of the most helpful factors in their lives. They found great comfort from religious communities especially from the value of relationships with others; being valued through a sharing of beliefs; and found participation in church religious activities important in enhancing feelings of self-worth. Some found that the religious help most useful was the practical and caring; and other supports included pastoral counseling, church programs, and small groups.

However, surveys showed that some people with mental illnesses in Christian congregations felt rejected; that some had been damaged by their experiences; that there was an inability by others to understand; that there were various forms of resistance within congregations; and that there were concerns about dangerousness and unpredictability. The surveys revealed that Christian congregations are uninformed on issues relevant to mental illnesses.

Further results from research showed that places of worship might be the only places where people with mental illnesses can meet socially, and be one of the few sources of information and support. The importance of friendships was stressed. The church and religious activities may be a considerable potential mental health resource towards psychiatric rehabilitation; that religious communities are channels in society of various sorts of support; and that compassion and kindness especially to the less fortunate are imperatives in most major religious traditions.

A lot of raising awareness and activity in contemporary Christianity has been reported in an earlier chapter. However, the results from my current survey suggest that a lot more needs to be done in order to help local congregations realize and understand that pastoral care and support is needed where there is mental illness.

This concludes the investigation into attitudes of members of Christian congregations into attitudes and understanding towards their members, but there are other aspects to examine.

Attitudes and spiritual beliefs
I continue by investigating whether or not respondents are influenced in their attitudes and understanding towards people with mental illnesses because of their basic spiritual beliefs, and furthermore, whether there is there a difference in results between the denominations.

Another section of the self-completion questionnaire listed fourteen statements in random order on a sheet of paper. Respondents were invited to indicate whether or not they personally agreed with the issue raised in each statement by ticking the "yes" or "no" box. The same format was used with each of the fourteen statements in determining whether or not respondents personally believed this to be their Church's teaching today. This allowed the respondents the freedom to identify their own opinion even if it did not coincide with what they believed to be their Church's teaching today.

For the purposes of analysis, each statement was allocated to one of four classifications. Classifications were labeled Humanity, Divine Intervention, Demonic Intervention, and Pastoral Care. Each statement was inspected and an attempt was made to identify underlying themes in order to place each statement within one of the classifications.

Percentages of majority responses to each of the fourteen components by the different denominations were collated, both of the personally held views of the respondents, and on what they believed to be their

Church's teaching today, and were compared statistically.

Humanity was the first classification examined in this section

Humanity
Each person with a mental illness is a unique person created by God
People with mental illnesses are not fully human
A person with a mental illness remains, in essence, a human being
People with mental illnesses have lost the essence of their humanity, that is, their reason

The results showed that there were significant differences between the denominations on responses to one of the components both in personally held views and what was believed to be their Church's teaching today, although the difference in percentages of respondents in each instance was small. The results are displayed below.

Each person with a mental illness is a unique person created by God
Personally held view
Anglican   89.30%   Roman Catholic   94.10%
Evangelical/Pentecostal   97.50%
Believed to be their Church teaching
Anglican   91.20%   Roman Catholic   94.50%
Evangelical/Pentecostal   98.20%

Of the next two listed components, there were very high percentages of respondents of all denominations, both in their personally held views and what is believed to be their Church's teaching today, on disagreeing with not being fully human, and agreeing with remaining in essence a human being. However, in disagreeing with the component displayed below, percentages of all respondents were slightly lower of personally held views than of what they believe to be their Church's teaching today.

People with mental illnesses have lost the essence of their humanity, that is, their reason
Personally held view
Anglican   83.70%   Roman   Catholic   84.30%
Evangelical/Pentecostal   84.70%
Believed to be their Church teaching
Anglican   89.50%   Roman   Catholic   85.10%
Evangelical/Pentecostal   87.60%

My literature research, reported in an earlier chapter, revealed that it was commonly held on theological grounds that being human implied having the faculty of reason. This theological thinking appears to be reflected in a small percentage of responses in my current survey.

Swinton argues that such a definition could imply that the more intelligent a person is, the more human they are with the inevitable corollary that the less intellectually equipped a person is, the less human they become. If insane people were deemed to have "lost their mind," it is possible that this line of reasoning could have had repercussions on attitudes towards these people, in resultant treatment of them as being less than human. In other words, as Swinton explains, "in adopting a rationalistic emphasis in one's definition of human beings, there is a real danger that people with severe mental illnesses can become dehumanized... if a person loses their reason, they, in a very real sense lose their humanity (Swinton, 1997a: 31).

Scull (1993) concedes that it must have been difficult not to draw the conclusion that in losing their reason, the essence of humanity, an insane person was not in a position to claim the right to be treated as a human being.

Pastoral Care: Mental Health

Davis (2000) gives an example of how it should be on a visit, in stating that he saw the patient as "one of God's children" and spent a lot of time talking with her "and believing in her worth as a human being" (Davis, 2000: 28).

A priest, who helped me set up a pastoral support group for those caring for a person with a mental illness, wrote his reflections.

> As a priest and shepherd in a town parish I come in contact with people with a mental illness. Sometimes this is through parish visitation of homes or sometimes in the local hospital. I always try and see them as a person with a mental illness, not as a mentally ill person. This is an important distinction. We do not say a broken leg person but a person with a broken leg, so also this should apply to a person with a mental illness. They are persons with beauty and dignity and who have rights. They need to be treated with the same care and attention as any other person. Persons with a mental illness have taught me a lot down the years. They have a deep spirituality and love and dependence on God. The courage, faith, and enduring hope they express, are always inspirational. They are always reassured when, after patient listening, I pray with them or pray over them. This helps calm their fears and anxieties. In the gospels, Jesus often meets with such people. He always treats them with dignity and compassion. He never fixes problems, but always heals. This is part of my vision in ministering to them. Father Eddie

Divine Intervention was the next classification examined in this section

Divine Intervention
Mental illnesses demonstrate rejection of persons by God because of the sins of their ancestors

Mental illnesses are punishments by God for wrongdoing
Mental illnesses are inflicted by God on people in order to test them

The results showed that there were no significant differences between the respondents of the denominations on their personally held views, nor on what they believed to be their Church's teaching today. Almost all the respondents personally disagreed, and also disagreed that it was their Church's teaching today, that mental illnesses were a sign of rejection, or punishment, or an infliction by God in order to test a person.

It is notable that there was a slight difference between personally held views of respondents and that which is considered by them to be their Church's teaching today, with respondents marginally more convinced in personally disagreeing than in disagreeing that it is their Church's teaching.

Demonic Intervention was the next classification examined in this section

Demonic Intervention
Mental illnesses are caused by evil spirits
People with mental illnesses are healed through exorcism
People with mental illnesses are possessed by the devil

The results showed that there were very significant differences between the denominations on responses of personally held views when disagreeing with three of the components, and also on responses when disagreeing with two of these components that this was believed to be their Church's teaching today. The results are displayed below.

Pastoral Care: Mental Health

Mental illnesses are caused by evil spirits
Personally held view
Anglican 99.20%   Roman Catholic 100.00%
Evangelical/Pentecostal 75.70%
Believed to be their Church teaching
Anglican 95.70%   Roman Catholic 96.10%
Evangelical/Pentecostal 80.40%

People with mental illnesses are healed through exorcism
Personally held view
Anglican 95.70%   Roman Catholic 97.10%
Evangelical/Pentecostal 77.50%
Believed to be their Church teaching
Anglican 92.50%   Roman Catholic 93.90%
Evangelical/Pentecostal 75.80%

People with mental illnesses are possessed by the devil
Personally held view
Anglican 99.60%   Roman Catholic 100.00%
Evangelical/Pentecostal 92.60%
Believed to be their Church teaching
Anglican 96.50%   Roman Catholic 95.50%
Evangelical/Pentecostal 92.00%

It is evident from these results that smaller percentages of the respondents of the Evangelical/Pentecostal fellowships personally disagreed, and disagreed that it was their Church's teaching today, with the content of the components, than of those of the respondents of the other two denominations.

The literature research, in earlier chapters, showed that from very early Christianity, one explanation of insanity was that good or evil spirits influenced people, and that the Christian practice of exorcism was advocated as a means of addressing the supposed demonic possession of insane people. From the early Church there has been tension between love and compassion and the battle of resisting the devil. Attitudes have been formed within this conflict. There was some attempt made to analyze mental derangement in the period of early Christianity, but a downside was the persecution of heretics becoming entangled with witchcraft, demonology and the phenomenon of insanity. The objective study of mental disorder developed intermittently with opposition to belief in witchcraft and demonic possession.

Koenig (2005) states that sometimes prejudices are rooted in religion such as belief that people with mental illnesses are being punished by God, or that they are possessed by the devil. He says that many religious groups around the world, including the United States, consider exorcism a valid method to rid a mentally ill person of their demons, but he argues that if demonic possession is responsible for the development of chronic mental illnesses, then exorcism should be an effective treatment. However, he insists that there is no evidence of this that no systematic research shows that exorcism is a successful treatment for severe mental illness, and that there is little evidence that religious beliefs predispose to the development of severe mental illnesses.

Pastoral Care was the final classification examined in this section

Pastoral Care
God loves all people equally including people with mental illnesses
People with mental illnesses are entitled to be given the same dignity and respect as other humans
People with mental illnesses merit special care because they are the poor in terms of status, finance and influence
Love of God shown by people to a person with a mental illness helps that person

The results showed that there were significant differences on responses to one component but only on personally held views and not what the respondents believe to be their Church's teaching today. The results are displayed below.

People with mental illnesses merit special care because they are the poor in terms of status, finance and influence
Personally held view
Anglican   76.10%   Roman   Catholic   72.50%
Evangelical/Pentecostal   63.10%
Believed to be their Church teaching
Anglican   68.30%   Roman   Catholic   68.80%
Evangelical/Pentecostal   64.60%

The largest diversity of opinion on all components in this section was on the responses to this component where the majority percentages of responses of each of the denominations were less than on any other component. The vast majority of all respondents agreed both in their personal views on the remaining three components and that they believe it to be the Church's teaching today.

Generally speaking, the investigation on this particular part of the examination of attitudes and understanding towards people with mental illnesses in Christian congregations in connection with spiritual beliefs, showed very small differences overall between denominations. Of the three denominations, it was the Anglican and Roman Catholic respondents who were much closer in agreement with their responses on all but one of the components where there were significant differences.

Pastoral support, states Davis (1953), is extremely important for both family and patient. In theory, Booth

(1953) believes that mental health is potentially strengthened by religious life because the Church emphasizes the dignity of each person and that God loves each individual no matter what gifts or talents one has.

Contrary to Freud's predictions, Koenig (1997) states that religion continues to play an important role in the lives of Americans of every age and questions why religion would persist in such a widespread manner if its effects on mental health were as damaging as suggested by Freud, Ellis and Watters, detailed in an earlier chapter. He concludes that in general, "devout religiousness and frequent involvement in both private and public religious activities are associated with better mental health." He recommends that patients should be encouraged to actively participate in a faith community as this may help reduce loneliness and isolation and "may reinforce religious beliefs that will help them to better cope with the stresses in their lives" (Koenig, 1997: 101, 121).

Koenig strongly feels that people of faith have a duty and responsibility to care for those who are troubled or in need, as the founders of every great religious tradition urge followers to care for the needy. He decrees, however, that when it comes to mental illness, much work remains to be done in educating faith communities about these illnesses and allaying concerns about dangerousness and unpredictability that prevent people of faith from reaching out to those persons, who, with severe mental illness, are the "most neglected of all those needing faith-based mental health services" (Koenig, 2005: 184).

Pattison (1993) concurs with the concept of pastoral care in terms of social justice and believes that there are others who think likewise. According to Pattison, there are authors who have expounded the belief that pastoral care is a means of fostering wholeness, that God is interested in both the public and private spheres of society, and to deny this is to deny a universal God. Pattison argues that there is a tendency towards mentally ill people being disadvantaged in society as a whole, as well as in the caring services. He refers to writers who have drawn on a worthy tradition that goes back to the Old Testament prophets that provokes questions about the social order. Social justice points the way in inviting Christians to consider the situation of mentally ill people, because the nature of social order is reflected in the suffering and condition of mentally ill people where those on the bottom are victims of indifference and injustice. In terms of power and influence in society, a place in social order and their needs being adequately met, "mentally ill people may be recognised as being among the poor and therefore have a claim on the interest and resources of the churches" because of two main elements of the Christian tradition, those of healing and of social concern and justice (Pattison, 1986: 35).

Having completed this section on attitudes and spiritual belief, there was a further dimension of interest regarding Christians and mental illnesses that I wished to investigate.

Attitudes on possible proneness to mental illnesses because of Christian faith

This part of the study covers an exploration into whether Christians, because of certain beliefs, possibly saw themselves as more prone to mental illnesses.

Respondents were presented with a set of twelve statements listed in random order within the same self-completion questionnaire. These covered a range of issues that might be thought to cause Christians to be more prone to mental illnesses. The respondents were asked to rate each statement on the five-point attitude scale, described and displayed in the previous chapter.

For the purposes of analysis, each statement was allocated to one of three classifications of Fear and Guilt, Spiritual Dimension, and Faith Intervention. Each statement was inspected and an attempt was made to identify underlying themes in order to place each statement within one of the classifications.

Firstly, percentages of majority responses to each of the twelve components were compared statistically. Secondly, responses to each of the twelve components were allocated to either neutral, agree, or disagree, as displayed in the previous chapter, collated and compared. This was to determine how much neutrality there was in responding, and whether this was linked with differences of opinion where definite responses were given.

Fear and Guilt was the first classification examined in this section

Fear and Guilt
Feeling unworthy in the sight of God can help cause mental illnesses
Christian people can develop mental illnesses because they are guilt ridden
Fear of God can cause mental illnesses
Fear of hell can cause mental illnesses

There was a significant difference between the denominations on their responses to one component of the Fear and Guilt classification, as displayed below.

Feeling unworthy in the sight of God can help cause mental illnesses

Anglican   43.70%   Roman   Catholic   41.20%
Evangelical/Pentecostal   55.30%

There were large differences in percentages of either agreeing or disagreeing on results to all of the components of this classification, as displayed below.

Feeling unworthy in the sight of God can help cause mental illnesses
neutral 20.10%   agree 45.20%   disagree 34.70%

Christian people can develop mental illnesses because they are guilt ridden
neutral 19.20%   agree 48.90%   disagree 31.90%

Fear of God can cause mental illnesses
neutral 23.40%   agree 21.20%   disagree 55.40%

Fear of hell can cause mental illnesses
neutral 24.80%   agree 31.10%   disagree 44.10%

Spiritual Dimension was the next classification examined in this section

Spiritual Dimension
Belief in evil spirits can exacerbate a mental illness
There are similarities between mental illnesses and spiritual/mystical experiences
Anyone can develop a mental illness whether Christian or not
A Christian's faith helps in sustaining a person who has a mental illness

Although there were differences between the denominations on the responses to the components of the Spiritual Dimension classification, they were not significant according to the statistical tests carried out.

However, the results showed that there was diversity in responding, particularly to two components, as displayed below.

There are similarities between mental illnesses and spiritual/mystical experiences
neutral 35.60%   agree 23.90%   disagree 40.50%

Belief in evil spirits can exacerbate a mental illness
neutral 15.90%   agree 56.50%   disagree 27.60%

Of the remaining two components, between seventy and ninety percent of respondents agreed that a Christian's faith helps in sustaining a person who has a mental, and almost all agreed that anyone can develop a mental illness whether Christian or not.

Faith Intervention was the final classification examined in this section

Faith Intervention
Having a faith helps in the prevention of mental illnesses
Christians are protected from mental illnesses because of their trust in God
Christians are less prone to mental illnesses because of their belief in an afterlife
Belief in God's love and care lessens the severity of a mental illness

With reference to the Faith Intervention classification, statistical tests gave rise to very significant differences between the denominations on the results of the responses to all four components. In each instance the respondents of the Anglican and Roman Catholic congregations were much closer in agreement than with those of the Evangelical/Pentecostal fellowships.

Also, there was much diversity in responses to each of the components as demonstrated in the examples displayed below.

Pastoral Care: Mental Health

Having a faith helps in the prevention of mental illnesses
neutral 21.60%   agree 49.00%   disagree 29.40%

Christians are less prone to mental illnesses because of their belief in an afterlife
neutral 25.50%   agree 21.30%   disagree 53.20%

Overall, two features are prominent from the results of responses to the components of the three classifications of Fear and Guilt, Spiritual Dimension and Faith Intervention. The respondents of the Evangelical/Pentecostal fellowships agreed to a greater extent that spiritual beliefs play a part in either preventing, protecting from, or made Christians less prone to, or help cause mental illnesses, than respondents of the other two denominations.

Secondly, the majority percentages of responses of Anglican respondents to nine of the twelve components were between forty and sixty-one percent; of the Roman Catholic respondents to nine were between forty-one percent to fifty-four percent; and of the Evangelical/Pentecostal respondents to eight were between thirty-two percent to fifty-nine percent, in either agreeing or disagreeing in each instance, signifying that similar percentages of respondents were either not in agreement or were unable to be definite in their opinion. Large percentages of sometimes up to approximately twenty-six percent of the respondents were uncertain about issues concerning mental illnesses and spirituality on seven of the twelve components; more than ten percent on a further three, and almost thirty-six percent on one. This suggests a diverse range of opinions by the Christian respondents or possible inability to give a definite response in many instances. The diversity in responding showed confusion over whether spirituality is interlinked with mental illnesses and if so, to what degree. Their real certainty was in knowing that anyone can develop a mental illness whether Christian or not.

The literature research provided some evidence on these issues. Koenig notes that like depression, anxiety and worry are widespread in America today, but reports that religious beliefs promise relief from anxiety, stress, and worry, though it is possible they might also increase anxiety through "arousing guilt over sins and worry about divine retribution." He explains that certain psychiatric disorders are characterized by obsessional preoccupation with a thought that evokes anxiety or guilt and such obsessions are often accompanied by compulsive, repetitive activities meant to relieve the anxiety. He says that "religious beliefs and activities nicely fit into the psychopathology of such persons," but he adds that the person is driven by deep anxieties rather than a love for God or holiness and it is their mental illness that drives these behaviors (Koenig, 1997: 63, 108).

Koenig believes that religious beliefs provide a worldview that is positive, coherent, optimistic, and caring, and that religion encourages people to turn to God, prayer, and their community. He suggests that feeling connected to, cared for, and loved by God, also helps to relieve loneliness, which more than anything else is often the life of someone with a mental illness. Religion helps people to know that they can still contribute and are valuable, and "by encouraging care for others provides a way for persons with mental illness to heal themselves" (Koenig, 2005: 138). Religion provides hope. However, he adds that a significant minority of psychiatric patients in the United States believes that religious factors are the cause of their illness, thus making it no longer tenable to ignore the role that religion plays in mental health care. Finally, Schade (1953) holds that people with mental illnesses may be found in almost any parish.

This chapter has shown that the Christian respondents seemed confident that people with mental illnesses should be supported but much less sure of whether this took place with their congregations. The next part of my study looked at some ways of trying to improve this situation in Christian congregations. The chapter includes added comment and discussion including testimonies of individuals, and concludes with recommendations. Could the implementing of these bring about enhanced understanding and increased pastoral support in this area of need?

Chapter 10

Addressing issues and integration of people with mental illnesses in Christian congregations

This chapter presents my investigation on two accounts. Firstly, I examine how Christians might address issues of mental illnesses within their congregations and in society in general. Secondly, I examine ways of how Christians might be involved in helping people experiencing the illnesses to be more personally integrated into their faith congregations.

A section of the questionnaire listed two sets of six statements placed in random order. The first set of statements made reference to how Christians might address issues of mental illnesses within their congregations and in society in general in order to raise awareness with the aim of increasing understanding and possible support for people with the illnesses. The second set made reference to possible ways of integration of people with mental illnesses into faith communities. Respondents were invited to rank the six statements in each of the sets, in order of priority, by numbering them one to six, the first choice one and second choice two, *et cetera*.

For the purpose of statistical analysis, the responses by the respondents to each of the six statements within addressing issues and similarly within integration were collated into rankings. Statistical tests were carried out on the percentages of rankings of the statements within each set of six. For the purposes of reporting the outcome of the tests, each set of six statements is introduced separately.

Addressing issues

The results of the tests to the set of six statements of Addressing Issues were examined, and rankings of statements placed in order of priority by the respondents, are displayed below.

Education is needed in Christian communities to increase awareness of the suffering and needs of people with mental illnesses and their families

Christian communities need to address any perceived stigma/fear attached to mental illnesses

More adequate training in pastoral ministry to people with mental illnesses and their families is needed for clergy/religious/laity

A Christian healing response to people with mental illnesses needs to include highlighting in the eyes of the public and the Government any lack of support

Christians working for justice for people with mental illnesses need to work alongside secular groups

People with mental illnesses need to be invited to participate in Church ministries

With reference to the six statements addressing issues, significant differences arose between the denominations on the ranking of responses to only one statement, that of adequate training in pastoral ministry to people with mental illnesses and their families. There were higher percentages of responses than the average by the respondents of the Evangelical/Pentecostal fellowships to this statement. Even so, there was no difference in the order of priority of rankings overall by the respondents of each of the different denominations.

The decision by the respondents to give top priority in addressing issues to the need for education showed that the Christian respondents appreciated that education is required to raise awareness of issues relevant to people with mental illnesses, and to provide information in order to improve in practice the other suggested ways of addressing issues.

These recommendations reinforce the earlier findings of uncertainty and diversity in responses, and reiterate mine when I recommended that education in both Church and the state sectors be undertaken to help remove prejudice and stigma (Hunneysett, 1998).

The need for education has been cited many times in my research in earlier chapters. Swinton stresses that understanding is the therapy and he believes that "*education* is fundamental to the task of overcoming congregational resistance" (Swinton, 1997a: 244).

Davis (2000), an ordained minister in Chicago, states that ignorance and misunderstanding often make people shun mentally ill persons and that pastors must reach out to these children of God and educate congregations to do the same, that mentally ill parishioners are just as in need of loving care as those suffering physical illness, and education is needed to counteract fear. Koenig (2005) adds that lack of knowledge is a huge barrier to feeling comfortable enough to get involved.

Address states that when a mental illness strikes a family it is devastating and because of misunderstandings, it can seem to be a humiliation that brings shame and isolation. There is profound suffering, and for family members, it would seem that the person they knew and loved, no longer exists, because a stranger appears to have taken over, but it is important for everyone to know that the family is not responsible for the illness. He adds that ignorance must not be tolerated, and together "we can break the stigma of mental illness and at the same time, I pray, lesson the rate of suicide" (Address, 2003: 35).

Puffer and Miller (2001), of the USA, present a proposal for how the church could become an agent of help to depressed elderly persons and their families. They suggest that the churches' current religious programming could be complemented with mental health promotion material. They propose such possibilities as educational workshops and weekend seminars with presentations in the form of videos and lectures with discussion groups. They admit to certain limitations in these proposals such as insufficient funds, over-worked pastoral professionals, and unmotivated lay leadership possibly due to a sense of inadequacy or being too busy, but suggest that assistance may be available from graduate level counseling students who may be willing to lead as part of their field experience. The authors assume the church communities care about the mental health of their elderly members, and they feel the church has a privileged position of ministry that they could extend to certain mental health concerns facing the elderly members of their congregation and community.

The next highest ranking of the need to address perceived stigma/fear implied not only the belief that stigma exists, a fact agreed on by a high percentage of respondents in earlier findings, but also that respondents in Christian communities felt strongly about addressing this.

This reinforces the findings reported in earlier chapters that there is stigma attached to mental illness in Christian congregations.

Woodward (1953) explains that because of stigma, most people are reluctant to reveal the extent of their guilt feelings and fears regarding mental problems, that the Church should be a place in which each person finds acceptance and recognition of true worth. Address (2003) agrees that there is a need to raise awareness of and reduce the stigma within congregations regarding individuals and families who experience mental ill health.

Stigma is enhanced by choice of language, as the Church of England guide reported earlier, reminding congregations to use language that does not belittle or exclude people. Davis reiterates this. He explains that, as leaders of the church, talking about "a real nut case" or someone being "looney" can have devastating effects on a person who is mentally ill and that we must avoid labels and ill-chosen expressions. He tells of a patient of whom no one from church visited when she was in hospital, that sometimes this happens because the patient is ashamed of being there and tells no one, "often the case because of the stigma of mental illness in our society" (Davis, 2000: 29). He is adamant that that these people need to know they are loved and supported because there is so much misunderstanding and stigma connected to mental illness.

I believe strongly that the label "mentally ill" takes away an individual's personhood and dignity and further to this, that people should not be described as "manics" or "schizophrenics" because these labels dehumanize them. People need to be given back their dignity. I was reminded of this in my place of work at the mental health day center.

"I am a nutter," was the opening statement by a disheveled-looking, middle-aged man sitting opposite

me. It was lunchtime on my first day at work. I had been told about Craig, a highly intelligent person who had developed schizophrenia later in life. He had had to give up work, and he lived alone, struggling to keep clean and fed, with little motivation for either.

"You are not a nutter," I insisted. "You are a person with a serious illness which happens to be called schizophrenia. You did not ask for it, but you got it. You suffer it, but you are not a nutter. I do not use that kind of language." He looked at me in surprise. I wondered, "Is he treated like a person in society or is his self-esteem so damaged that he no longer feels he has dignity, but feels a freak or, as he said, a nutter?"

"You know," I said later, to another member of staff in the art room, "each person in here is someone's mother, father, brother, sister, son or daughter." It could be my mother or daughter, I thought. These are real people, but they did not always feel as if the rest of the world saw them as such (Hunneysett, 2009).

When our teenage daughter was in hospital, the staff arranged for the young people to visit the local town hall to see a pop group. Elizabeth refused to go because they were being taken in a hospital bus with the hospital's name emblazoned on the outside. Elizabeth was terrified she would be seen by some of her peer group from her Catholic comprehensive school. Her peer group would know where she was. Such is the stigma.

The third choice of priority was of the need for more training in pastoral ministry to help people with mental illnesses and their families. This choice highlighted the importance the respondents of the Christian communities placed on training given regarding pastoral care where there is mental illness, particularly those of the Evangelical/Pentecostal communities.

This reflects the outcome of my research in an earlier chapter that demonstrated that although training content and resources in different denominational Colleges varied, and there was evidence of raising awareness and concern for mental illness across all three denominations, there was a conclusion that more needed to be done in the training of ministers in this area of pastoral ministry especially in view of the comments by the respondent of a Roman Catholic College and by the leaders of Evangelical/Pentecostal fellowships.

Howe reports of a minister in America explaining that he received the best theological training available, "but it was education for theological study and teaching and not training for the work of ministry;" that the clergy's criticism is of an overemphasis on subject matter and not enough on people, relationships and needs (Howe, 1953: 239). Howe adds that a part of training should be working with people. Davis (2000) agrees that most pastors have not been trained in working with mentally ill people, and Koenig (2005) insists that in the United States, educating clergy about such issues is necessary to decrease negative perceptions that are even held by many clergy after seven years of training.

Of the statements of Addressing Issues, it was only after having given priority to increasing their own understanding, addressing the stigma, and increased training in pastoral ministry to people with mental illnesses and their families, did the respondents choose the points of highlighting any lack of support to the general public and Government, and working alongside secular groups. The results implied that the priority of the respondents was to improve attitudes amongst all members before finally concentrating on involving people with mental illnesses in Church ministries.

Integration

The results of the tests to the set of six statements of Integration were examined. Rankings of statements placed in order of priority by the respondents are displayed below.

People with mental illnesses need befriending in Christian communities

People with mental illnesses and their families should be offered practical support by the Christian community

Members of Christian communities need to make a point of inviting people with mental illnesses to the communities' social activities

Visitation to the homes of people with mental illnesses to be undertaken by clergy/religious or authorized lay person as part of pastoral ministry

Christian community drop-in centers need to be made available to people with mental illnesses

Members of Christian communities should invite people with mental illnesses to share in prayer with them

With reference to the six statements of integration, there were significant differences between the denominations on the rankings of responses to two of the six statements. The respondents of both the Evangelical/Pentecostal and Anglican congregations ranked higher than the average that people with mental illnesses need befriending with the

Evangelical/Pentecostal respondents giving the higher ranking of the two. Respondents of the Roman Catholic congregations gave a higher ranking than the average to the statement of visitation in homes. Of the other two denominations, the Anglican respondents had a higher ranking than the Evangelical/Pentecostals on this statement.

The statistical tests showed that there was a slight variation in the order of priority of ranking by the denominations. The Anglican respondents ranked befriending and offering practical support as joint first priorities and sharing in prayer as sixth choice. The Roman Catholic respondents ranked offering practical support as their highest priority and, like the Anglican respondents, placed sharing in prayer sixth. They also ranked visitation of homes as a third priority whereas the Anglican respondents placed it fourth. The Evangelical/Pentecostal respondents gave the highest ranking to befriending people with mental illnesses and placed visitation of homes, sixth. However, in spite of these slight differences, there was little difference between the percentages on the ranking of the statements by respondents as a whole, with befriending and practical support given much more priority than the other four suggested ways of integration.

The decision by the respondents to give top priority within Integration to the need to befriend people with mental illnesses indicated that the respondents understood that people with mental illnesses are not always able to join in community activities but that it is important to support them. This was reinforced by the second priority of offering practical support followed thirdly by inviting people with mental illness to the social activities. Putting these choices higher than providing drop-in centers and praying with them is a sign of the recognition by the respondents that it is important that a holistic approach is undertaken when helping to integrate people with mental illnesses into Christian congregations, that relationships are important to their mental wellbeing, and this reinforces earlier findings that a high percentage of respondents agreed there is a need for more embracing attitudes towards people with mental illnesses.

Interestingly, the Roman Catholics placed visitation third in priority and the Anglicans fourth but those of the Evangelical/Pentecostal fellowships placed it last. Possibly, with smaller communities, there is not felt the same need for personal contact as expressed by the Roman Catholic respondents particularly. On the other hand, the fact that the Evangelical/Pentecostals placed praying with people with mental illnesses higher than those of the other two denominations possibly reinforces the stronger views that they hold on links between mental illnesses and spirituality.

The top priority of befriending reflects the message of the video reported in an earlier chapter that included resources. It also runs parallel to the theme presented by Swinton, about befriending.

The task of the Christ-like friend is not to <u>do</u> anything for them, but rather to <u>be</u> someone for them, someone who understands and accepts them as persons: someone who is <u>with</u> and <u>for</u> them in the way that God is also <u>with</u> and <u>for</u> them; someone who reveals the nature of God and the transforming power of the Spirit of Christ in a form that is tangible, accessible, and deeply powerful (Swinton, 2000: 143).

Koenig (2005) states that support from religious communities is vital and cites the Interfaith Compeer staff in America, a local organization helping adults and children with mental illness, believing, according to their website, that "friendship is priceless." Davis (1953) emphasizes that we can all be compassionate friends and listeners, while Swinton believes that the friendships Jesus had were always personal and primarily aimed at regaining the dignity and personhood of the individuals whom society had rejected and depersonalized. He adds that awareness of the transcendent love of God is "mediated through, and experienced in, temporal love, offered in loving relationships" (Swinton, 1997b: 24).

Bruder (1953) agrees that visiting the family after seeing the patient in hospital, helps to break down the stigma associated with mental illness, and gives the family a chance to verbalize fears and guilt associated with the hospitalization. Schade (1953) agrees that the families usually appreciate the opportunity to voice these feelings and thoughts even if they have not sought the pastor's counsel, and he suggests maintaining contact with the patient's family. He believes that prayers with the sick person's family not only benefit the ill person but the family themselves to prepare for possible months of recovery when patience, love and understanding will be needed.

Addressing issues and integration

The results of the percentages of addressing issues, and of integration of people with mental illnesses into congregations, were looked at together as a measure of determining overall priority. The four statements with the highest percentages of rankings by statistical analysis arising from all twelve statements are displayed below in order of descending priority of the average percentage of ranking.

Education is needed in Christian communities to increase awareness of the suffering and needs of people with mental illnesses and their families

People with mental illnesses need befriending in Christian communities

People with mental illnesses and their families should be offered practical support by the Christian community

Christian communities need to address any perceived stigma/fear attached to mental illnesses

The highest ranking of the twelve statements was that education is needed and this was substantially higher than the others. The next three rankings were of responses to the statements on befriending, offering practical support to people with mental illnesses, and addressing the perceived stigma/fear attached to mental illnesses. The three denominations were in total consensus that these four issues were top priority of the twelve statements responded to. These results demonstrate that the Christian respondents appreciate that in order to support, education, above all else, is needed first in order to raise awareness of issues relevant to people with mental illnesses.

The importance of these four points was highlighted many times in the research detailed in earlier chapters.
Koenig (1997) puts forward three natural mechanisms by which religion might promote mental health. Firstly, through a system of beliefs and mental attitudes; secondly, through increased support and promotion of interaction with others; and thirdly, by emphasizing a

focus on others and on a power higher than the self. He recommends that members of the congregation should be directed and motivated to reach out to those in need both within and outside the church, and that pastors will require the support of their lay members in order to meet these needs.

For example, I met a married couple at a Catholic National Conference in 2006. The husband was in our very small mental health group, the aim of which was to look at ways of how parishes can make a positive difference to families where there is a mental illness. He told his story of how he had become mentally ill and had to give up his job, and was unable to go to church. Eventually visits from church stopped because he was told that they could not cope with his pain. Consequently, he and his wife were left feeling very isolated. A parishioner, on hearing of the weeks and months of their difficult life at home and of all the suffering, suggested to his wife that she leave him. Yet Richardson (1953) states that it is through the Church's ministry that a sick person is transported from a sense of loneliness into a realm of hope and trust. Later, the husband was able to return to church through the help of a kind neighbor who offered to walk with him.

A positive example is revealed through Ted's story. He was one of the clients allocated to my care at the mental health day center where I worked. He was helped through the kindness of a church leader and the acceptance of some parishioners.

Ted was a jocular sort of person, always talking, giving his opinion and joining in the laughter. It was noticeable one morning when he seemed unusually subdued.

"And how are you today, Ted?" I asked, over a coffee break.

"Today is the anniversary of when my mother died. I still miss her even after all these years."

"I'm sorry, Ted. Have you no relatives?"

"No, none. No brothers or sisters. I have nobody. My mother looked after me. I became so ill after she died. I used to sit in the park a lot. Sunday was the worst day. There was nowhere to go. We even had our own bench, you know. You would see the same people sitting there, day after day. Eventually, I was picked up by social services and ended up in the mental hospital. I was ill, you see."

Later that day, I met up with Ted again.

"Where are you now, Ted? Where do you live?"

"I am in a hostel now with my own room. It's very nice. Others are there who have been in the hospital. The staff support us if we need help."

"So how did you recover? What helped you this far?" *Ted looked at me.*

"I'll tell you." *He told me his story.*

"There was this vicar from one of the council estates, who used to come into the hospital, and he used to stop and chat to me. He said that when I was discharged, I could visit him. So I did. I started going to his church and eventually into the hall for coffee after the service. I only have one friend whom I visit once a week, so it was somewhere to go. Two or three of the women were very friendly to me, and kind. I started helping with coffee mornings. Then I was invited on to the parish council. I joined a Bible study group as well. Our vicar invites me to his Christmas dinner each year. So I always have *somewhere to go on Christmas day. You know, Edna, I found Jesus again with going there. I'm happy now. We are going to have a new church built and I am helping with the fund raising."* Ted had regained his dignity and self-respect because he had been accepted as he was. He had found Christ through the love and support of the vicar and some of the congregation (Hunneysett, 2009).

Counseling is another example of support that carers of people with mental illnesses may find particularly helpful, and likewise, people with mental illnesses.

Davis speaks of Mary whose faith had always been an important component of her recovery, and that her psychologist had to be "someone who was understanding of the importance of God in her life" (Davis, 2000: 47).

To have a counselor of the same basic spirituality, I believe, is doubly beneficial, as I discovered when I was a broken carer and was "rescued" by a nun who freely gave me her time in hourly sessions for eight weeks, eighteen months into our daughter's illness. After our daughter's relapse two years later, I benefited further from counseling.

The Saturday morning following Elizabeth's attempted overdose, I was sitting after Mass in church quietly weeping when Father Desmond came over to me. I told him through my tears of Elizabeth's illness. He was new to the parish and did not know her.

"I will come and see her."

"Thanks, Father," I whispered. Later that morning, he arrived at our house. Elizabeth and I sat with him in the kitchen. She looked pale and drawn

with dark shadows under her eyes through lack of sleep. She told him how she felt. It was obvious that she was in a severe depression. He did not know what to say, but I felt he showed compassion by coming and listening and I appreciated that.

Three days later, he found me again in church.

"I have thought about you and Elizabeth all weekend. I could not sleep because her face kept coming into my mind. I do not know how to help, Edna, but maybe a woman will be better than me for you. I asked a fellow priest who knows of a Catholic counselor who would be more than happy to see you if you would like to talk with her." He gave me a name and number. I thanked him for this information and later, contacted the lady in question who lived quite close by. Somehow it helped me to know that she was a trained counselor and a Catholic. I went a number of times to see her. She was quite happy for me to go irregularly when I felt the need. It helped greatly to know that I could do this when desperate. I felt better for seeing her as she helped me lift my low self-esteem, a side effect of the stress I was under (Hunneysett, 2009).

Pastoral support groups are another means of supporting either carers or people with the illnesses.

As far back as the 1950s, Maves (1953) speaks of there being an awakening interest in, and the importance of, working more effectively in groups in which pastoral work is enhanced, and in which individuals are enabled to support one another. He describes groups as constantly in progress and dynamic, within which, are provided experiences of acceptance, understanding, and respect, that allows participants to express verbally negative as well as positive feelings. He feels that perhaps the development of Christian nurture groups may be one of the main contributions the Church can make to health but that they must be person and need centered. Woodward likewise believes that people who have been in a mental hospital or even not hospitalized but experiencing mental ill health "need opportunities to participate in some group in order to complete their recovery," and that a minister can prepare a group by explaining that there is no reason to stigmatize such a person (Woodward, 1953: 152).

Understanding and support at grass roots level is evident in the self-help pastoral support groups reported in an earlier chapter. For example, Father Joseph and I initiated a carers pastoral support group in the 1990s for those caring for people with mental illnesses. Over the years, carers come and go. Sister Deirdre, a parish worker, supported us from the beginning and continued to do so after Father Joseph was moved to another parish and no longer able to attend. Sister is not able to join us now but she told us how she felt about the years with the carers.

"It has been a real blessing and a privilege to have been part of your group. I have found it so enriching and I have learnt so much from each one of you. I certainly gained and received far more than I gave." Sister Deirdre

I had found no help when our daughter was first ill, but when she had her relapse, the counselor, to whom the priest had referred me, was there for me, as was our carers pastoral support group.

On the last Thursday evening of the month, I drove to St. Thomas More's church and went into the small hall. I sat down and looked at the lighted candle and

the open Bible that Sister Deirdre had placed on the table ready for us. She entered the hall.

"How are things with you, Edna?"

"Not so good." She sat down beside me. Soon there were six of us seated in a semicircle with Father Joseph who had joined us. He welcomed everyone and briefly explained the format, the sharing of Scripture and whatever else people might like to say arising from this sharing. Often we tried to see it in the context of our present day circumstances. He emphasized the confidentiality; the listening, and that no one need feel under pressure to speak

We are light-hearted at times and even have a laugh in spite of tears. Some individuals are too emotional even to contribute verbally, but somehow draw comfort and strength from the sharing. We know we are not alone in our pain. We understand one another and are no longer isolated. I feel supported in this atmosphere and receive consolation from the sharing and empathy. We hear of God's love for us, which we find through each other. Father Joseph draws the meeting to a close with a short prayer. I come home refreshed and strengthened a little and more ready to face the difficult days ahead (Hunneysett, 2009).

I met Margaret when we began our pastoral support group for carers. She attended each meeting for a number of months with her mother-in-law, but never spoke. Eventually, she started to contribute verbally, and after time, came on her own. She told me her story.

Chris and I married with nuptial Mass. We had a little girl, and about three years later, a baby boy. Both were christened in the Catholic Church. While they were still very young, Chris took ill but I did not understand what was happening. It was a terrible time and we did not get a diagnosis that it was manic depression, now bipolar, until much later.

I was on a new estate and there was no Catholic primary school near. It took me all my time to get to church. A priest came to our house to tell me that Chris had to stop ringing the parish priest, as he did not want to be disturbed. Chris had been doing this because of his mania. I went to ask the priest, who knew of our situation, if there was any help in getting our first child to the nearest Catholic primary school, some distance away, as neither of us drove a car then. I got no help.

A health visitor got our little daughter into a local non-catholic school early, as I was ill coping with Chris, and my little girl, and boy under two years old, and she was worried about my health. No one came to visit although we kept going to church. The kids never went to Catholic schools because I did not have time to focus, and my family did not understand about Chris. I struggled, and Chris struggled in and out of hospital. So the kids never received the sacraments and it fills me with great sadness to this day and I pray that it will come right even though they are adults now. A neighbor who worked at the hospital told all the neighbors that Chris had been in hospital and they name-called Chris and the kids and shouted things at him in the street. We sold the house and moved in with his parents because of that.

I searched and searched for a carers group but could not find any. I wanted to talk and relate to others who had experienced what I had been through and how important God is in my life. When in the depths of despair, I know God has his hand on my shoulder although it did not always feel like that. To be in a Christian group is such a great help, just to be able to come and confide and also to know it is confidential. It has got me through the worst days of my life. I knew you always made sure someone would be there even if just one. I knew I could pick up the phone and you would always be there even if I never did. I used to cry out loud to God. Why? Why? I cannot go on anymore. He always sent the people, others, not just you. I wanted to talk and then when I came to the group I couldn't because I knew I would cry. Margaret

Margaret insists it is her faith that has kept her going and she has a great sense of humour. She stopped coming for a while and eventually I met with her in a parish hall after a Healing Mass. She told me she had been seeing a psychiatrist as she had become so ill. She has found great comfort from Healing Masses and prayer with people. She started to come regularly again to the pastoral support group and still attends.

There was another area of pastoral care that I was concerned about. I had encountered many people with mental illnesses during the course of my studying, and at venues at which I had spoken publicly. I spent many months thinking about these people. I prayed for guidance.

I decided that I would initiate a pastoral support group for people with mental illnesses, to be available if needed. I contacted Father Bill, chaplain to St. Luke's mental hospital, who offered his support. Father Bill insisted that we let those with the illnesses decide on the length and frequency of meetings, and format. We would empower them.

I had Mary utmost in mind as she had already made contact with me and attended our carers group on one occasion. We met and chatted on another occasion at her request, and I was aware of her suffering and feelings of neglect by her church community. Mary is widowed. She has four young adult children. She told me her story.

Looking back, I realise that I have had a mental illness for as long as I can remember. My family thought of me as being moody and very bad-tempered. I had my first bout of serious depression when I was seventeen and at the sixth form college. I became a different person, always very tired, stayed in bed for long periods of the day, and often absent from college. I was very anti the music teacher whom I saw as being very arrogant and not good for my self-esteem; so I was often rude to him. I isolated myself at home by spending hours in my bedroom, easily upset, often angry and irritable, had difficulty in communicating, and when in the kitchen looked at the knives and thought how easy it would be to pick one up and kill myself; also did the same with tablets.

Obviously I was extremely unhappy with myself, confused, wanted to be helped but did not know how. It was clear to my parents that something was wrong and they kept questioning me.

"What is the matter? What is wrong?" My older brother, John, whom I was very close to, also asked because my parents thought that I was more likely to tell him. How could I when I myself did not know? They were very worried about me. Eventually Dad took me to see our doctor. My mother would not go as she said that Dad would be listened to, another indicator of how worried they were, as I usually went on my own and never with my Dad. My doctor said that I was recovering from influenza even though I had not been ill.

A few months later when watching television, I saw a programme about depression and recognised myself and told my parents who had also watched the programme. However, we did not do anything about it as by this time I was beginning to pick up and I refused to talk about it for a very long time. I think I was ashamed of how I had been. Obviously, my college work suffered and I did not do as well as I should have done at my exams, but I managed to go on and qualify as a teacher.

Pastoral Care: Mental Health

Initially, it didn't affect me spiritually, as thanks to my primary school and the nuns there, as well as my parents and my grandmother, I had a deep faith in God and constantly turned to Him and Mary for help and support. I spent a lot of time praying and I am certain that this is what kept me going over the years. I was affected following my diagnosis of having a mental illness. Having been absent from work as a result of the illness, for several months at a time, I found that I could not continue to work and was allowed to retire on grounds of ill health. As a courtesy, I telephoned the head to inform her and was shocked at her response.

"Oh, you are ill then!" Not the expected response as I had worked closely with this person for several years.

My spiritual difficulties began during the year I was off work prior to retiring. During that year, apart from one occasion, none of my colleagues visited me. Several of them lived nearby. Apparently, when they saw Kevin, my husband, or my friend, Catherine, they asked after me. Both Kevin and Catherine said to call in or telephone me and not to worry because, if I did not feel up to the contact, I would say so. My ex-colleagues did not make the effort and it was as though I was a different Mary now that I had a mental illness. As I worked in a Roman Catholic primary school where we taught Christian values, this neglect was difficult to understand. As Christians, surely they should have been there for me?

I usually played the organ at Saturday evening Mass but was no longer able to. I contacted the clergy to let them know and said that when I well enough to play again, I would be in touch. I had been finding it difficult to attend Mass during that year because I felt unacceptable to members of the congregation. I knew that my body language discouraged people from approaching me. That was not what I wanted. I did not wish to have a conversation but would have appreciated a touch on my arm and a smile to reassure me that I was acceptable in spite of my illness. Not much to hope for, I thought. The whole of the Mass was a constant reminder to me that I was not experiencing the love, support, and care, that Jesus taught all of us to give. Selective Christianity! We will apply it to well known members of the community and to those who have an obvious physical illness, but we will avoid those whom we find difficult to be with and those who have a mental illness. Regularly during Mass, I had a very strong urge to stand up and shout out.

"What about me? Where do I fit in to all of this?" I stopped attending Mass. This upset my husband because he knew the importance of my faith to me, but he fully understood why I stopped going.

I was further hurt when the clergy did not visit me. There was obviously a problem. Eventually, I plucked up courage to ask Kevin if the clergy asked about me. It was no surprise to hear the answer.

"No." It was not as though I was a stranger to them. I needed not only support from my family, but also from my parish family. I felt so alone, and the neglect reinforced my low self-esteem and sense of worthlessness. At times, I was very angry about my situation. It was difficult enough to have a mental illness without the lack of spiritual and community support. I decided that I needed to deal with it. I approached a curate in the parish who was known to me as not only did he visit my classroom but I also spoke to him at the cathedral. On one occasion, I offered to speak with him about my experience of mental illness because I was confident that he would meet many like me, over the years. The offer was not taken up. My chat with him was very damaging to me and if anything, made matters worse. He kept saying the same thing to me.

"You only had to ask for help." He could not understand that it is impossible to do that. It is very important to have the need recognised, and to be approached. It became apparent to me that I was upsetting him and I backed off. I kept apologising and left. There was no help or support given.

Some time later, I approached the bishop who was happy to talk, but said that awful phrase.

"You have to make allowances. People do not understand." I have a question.

"Why? Why do I have to make allowances? Are they frightened that I might suddenly turn on them and harm them physically? I am the one who is ill and in need of help."

Obviously, none of these experiences did anything to stop my resentment for my parish community. They fed it. Over time I recognise that I needed spiritual input as well as contact with my faith community. Having recognised this, I met with the bishop on several occasions and explained what I thought was needed for myself and others like me. He did not understand that I was not able to do this myself. I had the idea but it required others to put it in place. I gave up. The only good thing to come out of the chats with the bishop was meeting Edna.

Having given up, the support I needed arose. It took years to arrive at this point and was such a relief. I cannot recall how many years it took but our group was worth waiting for. The mix of spiritual input, sharing of our lives, and the social time that we have is very important to me. It is my only contact with my faith community, as I still cannot attend Mass. I attend other churches now and again, but unfortunately, my negative experience with my parish community has resulted in my feelings been transferred to all Roman Catholic communities.

How different it would have been had I had the experience of Christian love and caring that my husband had during his life with terminal cancer. He was very aware of the different treatment that he received from his colleagues (Kevin taught in a Roman Catholic secondary school), and also from our parish community and clergy. He was very hurt for me, and my observations of his good experience just fuelled my anger, hurt, and feeling of being rejected/unwanted.

Edna Hunneysett

My experience makes it very clear that support is needed. All of the time I have been aware of all those who have suffered in silence and needed support from their church. Perhaps they have left and nobody has noticed.

"You have to make allowances. People don't understand." Therefore, parishioners need to be helped to understand; so some sort of education is required. They also need to know that they can help just by acknowledging a person with a nod or smile or touch or a combination. It is that easy. Do it to everybody and what a lot of good feeling will be generated. The clergy need to be educated as they often meet parishioners with a mental illness, but may avoid them because they can be very difficult to be with. I think that we are all aware of that.

For those who need more, then a support group like ours could be good for them, spiritual, mutually supportive, social occasions. There are support groups out there, but I felt strongly that the Church should be able to support its own and a good beginning is a group, as members begin with two things in common, mental illness and belief. Groups should be open to accepting a person who wants to become more involved in supporting those who need it. The clergy should visit a group from time to time even if unable to make a commitment to regular meetings.

Bishops need to be pro-active and encourage support. I suppose education should begin with them. They in their turn should make sure that the clergy of the diocese should attend an awareness day where they will, hopefully, gain an understanding of living with mental illness, as a sufferer and as a carer. All of them need to be aware that support requires flexibility. There is no one right way. Support may be one to one at home by priest, deacon or sympathetic parishioner, being accompanied to Mass, or a support group. I envisage there could be many of these so it may be necessary for parishioners, able to empathise, to help establish a new group. Mary

Mary reinforces much that has already been revealed in the literature and research detailed in earlier chapters. She felt the neglect of ex-colleagues, that she was unacceptable in church, the lack of love, care, and support from the parish family, hurt by clergy not visiting, alone, low in self-esteem and feelings of worthlessness, the importance of having needs recognised, and she needed spiritual input. The priorities my survey highlighted are also amongst those she suggests of education of ministers and laity. Mary needed friendship and spiritual support. She felt she was treated differently when compared with her husband who was well supported through his cancer. The stigma needs addressing.

Koenig (2005) relates a similar experience in Minnesota of a lady whose son was diagnosed with schizophrenia and at around the same time her mother was diagnosed with cancer. The lady said that she received not a fraction of support, nothing, from her faith community and friends for her son in comparison to the visits and prayers for her mother. She says that they did not even ask how he was. It was totally different.

A few months after Father Bill and myself had established the pastoral support group, another lady, Catherine, contacted me. She came to talk to me for an hour, confidentially, having read my book. I offered the pastoral support group but she declined. However, after a week, she contacted me again and said she would like to come. Catherine is married. Her husband is not a Catholic. They have four young adult children. This is her story.

"All over the world, the Spirit is moving, all over the world as the prophets said it would be, all over the world there's a mighty revelation of the glory of the Lord as the waters cover the sea."

When it was suggested to me that I might benefit from joining a mental health support group in the diocese, my first reaction was the thought, thank you but no thank you. I had experienced a re-occurrence of clinical depression and anxiety, a condition with similar features of other mental illnesses including: exhaustion, feelings of isolation, thoughts like "I don't want to die but I have no energy to function, breathe, think, or live." I thought to myself that the last thing I needed was the company of people who felt like I did. I feared this would make me feel more ill and depressed. I imagined a group of people focused on problems and illness and I certainly did not want to be part of a group like that. I told my kind friend that I would let her know. In time, after feeling a bit more lost and desperate, I decided to give the group a try, and I thank God that I did because I have discovered a place of refuge, strength, grace, and healing.

"For where two or three meet in my name, I am there among them" (Mt. 18:20).

Why does the group work? The group works because we believe and experience the Holy Spirit is invited and present with us. How? There is a high level of trust amongst the participants that has developed through time spent in prayer, meditation on the Word of God from the scriptures, and sharing of individual experiences without fear of negative judgements or criticism. Could the group develop? Yes. We want to share what we have discovered in the hope and belief that other small groups could come together using a simple format "K I S S" "Keep it Safe and Simple."

Safe: even among some Christians, there is a stigma of mental ill health and some of us felt we do not want to be identified as attending "a support group" unless we decide to make a self-disclosure, if and when appropriate. Within the group, confidentiality is an essential element of our relationship. The sharing together of heart, mind and spirit

Pastoral Care: Mental Health

must be within a safe place without fear of personal or family information being discussed outside of the group and the sacred space created by God's presence within. While the number is flexible, we all felt that small is easier to cope with, in allowing each person to feel at ease and able to speak if they want to do so. There is no pressure to talk. Each person is giving a valuable contribution by being "present." Quietness or silence is perfectly acceptable.

Simple: an opening prayer is offered. We open in prayer remembering we belong to God's family and He is present with us. We share each other's company and tasty tea and cake. We share a scripture reading and meditation. Following reflections, a closing prayer is offered with thanks to God for all we have received in our encounter with Him and each other. The meeting lasts for one hour and thirty minutes. Some attend weekly and others fortnightly. This arrangement has proved to be manageable for us all, with the usual exceptions on occasions, and gives regard to energy and concentration levels within the group.

What are the benefits? Each person in the group has reported dramatic, positive health effects of our time together in mutual giving, sharing, and receiving, within a God-centred environment. Together we thank all who have made this group possible. My personal benefits: I reluctantly left a career I enjoyed, five years ago, following a long and complex illness of severe anaemia. (Mental illness often accompanies physical ill health). Thanks to this wonderful group of people, I am no longer ashamed that sometimes I get sick because I realise I am how God created me for His purpose. When I have health and energy, I work therapeutically and creatively in ways that are meaningful to me. I am a director of a charitable trust A.R.C. and I develop my creative arts project. I try to compensate my family and friends for the times I have not been there for them. The rainbow is my favourite symbol from the bible signifying joy, hope and love.

Creativity is an integral part of our humanity and a gift of the Holy Spirit of God. "Your light must shine in people's sight, so that seeing your good works, they may give praise to your Father in heaven" (Mt. 5:16). I enjoy writing, singing and playing with my beloved grandson, Frankie.

The group has helped me to develop a greater attitude of gratitude. When a mother gets sick, it has consequences for all of the family. I would like to thank all of my family for their love and patience with me especially my husband Samuel (means sent from God) and he was. Sam has upheld me and loved me when I could not love myself or stand on my feet. I thank God that despite many periods of illness, I have more than my share of happiness, through the deep love I receive from God, my family and my friends, which includes my new friends in the pastoral group, and for this I am always grateful.

Our Lady of Mental Peace, pray for us (prayer cards available). Catherine

This group had the support of Father Bill. Our Bishop expressed an interest in participating and came to one of our meetings to experience it, and suggested we have a write-up in our diocesan newspaper, anonymously, if that is what we wished. Catherine mentions that there is still stigma among Christians, but since participating in the pastoral group, she no longer feels ashamed. Not only did she do the write-up for the diocesan newspaper, but also, with great courage, she put her name to it knowing that her extended Catholic family and parishioners would discover her "secret."

When I mentioned to Margaret about the pastoral support group for those with mental illnesses, she asked if she could come. She appreciates so much the benefits from being with others in a prayer-filled atmosphere where there is confidentiality, respect, and care towards one another. Margaret attends whenever her family commitments allow.

I invited another lady, Kay, whom I had kept in touch with and who came in the early days to our carers pastoral group, although she was not a carer but suffered herself, but ceased coming as she felt that she did not quite fit in. Kay, single and retired, declined initially to attend this pastoral group for people with the illnesses, but eventually decided to participate. She told me her story.

> The trouble is I cannot encourage people, as life seems such a burden to me, just going on living. I so much want to die and be out of it. I start each day with a prayer and tell myself if God wants me to live another day then I will do the best I can. I have lost all faith in the Church. I believe others support me but its blind faith. I go to Mass every week because I play the organ. I go in the week when a friend needs a lift or something, but again, I struggle with so much of what is done and said there. It makes so little sense in terms of the God I trust in and Jesus whose life I want to follow.
>
> I first experienced depression when my mother died suddenly in January 1989. Then I was teaching at a sixth form college. When she died, my life seemed very empty. After the funeral, I returned to school, but eventually, I had to go to the doctor and was given some pills, but no time off. After developing bulimia and losing a lot of weight, I went into St. Luke's mental hospital. A priest was very good and brought me Holy Communion every day until I was allowed to go out to Mass. After two months, I was discharged and was supposed to see a clinical psychologist but this never really happened, as there were long waiting lists. I was made redundant in 1992 and felt very upset at the way it happened and the lack of any concern from the senior staff of what I had been led to believe was a caring Catholic community.

> My best help came from a bereavement counselor, whom I met at a Eucharistic ministers meeting, who offered help. Although people can be sympathetic when they know you are suffering, I do not think that the church community knows how to help except for promising to pray, and I do not know how to ask. I think the groups you have set up sound marvelous, just to be with people without feeling a nuisance. Kay

On her second participation with the group, Kay commented on how lovely it was to be with people where she can truly be herself and not be judged. She continues to attend fortnightly, distance being part of the problem as she lives in another town. Kay had been very touched by the priest frequently bringing her Holy Communion when in the mental hospital.

Davis (2000) reminds ministers that what a patient needs is not advice but to experience in a visit, God's unconditional love. Howe states that "the Church and its ministry can be one of the most powerful influences of mental health" (Howe, 1953: 252), and Hiltner (1953) believes that the difficulty that has brought a person into hospital has also made his religious need more acute. According to Bruder (1953), one of the most helpful contributions to increase the patient's self-esteem is when a representative of the community, particularly clergy, makes a friendly visit.

Feelings of higher self-worth when relying on religion confirm research of a survey in America detailed in an earlier chapter, and Koenig (2005) affirms that clergy deliver an enormous amount of mental health services to needy persons and families that are seldom recognized by mental health professionals. He states that estimates of unmet need are particularly high in African American communities, and clergy are often a key source of mental health services in minority communities.

Father Bill was given a parish at the other end of the diocese and we no longer see him, but before he went, he told me how he had gained his understanding in this area of pastoral care.

> Ideas are learnt through the media, negative, fear, violence. You learn through contact with people and I think you can be trained. For example, do not say pull yourself together. There are basic rules, good guidelines, to walk with people with mental illness. Pastoral studies were very strong as I did a theology/ministry degree when training.
> My first contact was when I was asked to visit a lad with schizophrenia and I was apprehensive as I did not know what I was going to face, but I thoroughly enjoyed visiting and have done so many times since.
> I gained insight from groups and hospital, but more so in groups. More severe in hospital but still learning from them and learnt a great deal from them but a bit more defensive, but in groups, more open. Best way to learn is to have contact with them and let them tell you and if they get angry, just let them, and if they want to talk about Church, let them. Empower the people in the groups. For example, what you want, the decision is yours. Father Bill

Davis (2000) reiterates this in saying that people who are depressed do not want to be told to snap out of it and that comments such as these come from ignorance. Bruder (1953) states that unless what is being done for a patient in the name of religion reflects an acceptance of him or her as a person, shows something of an understanding of the suffering, and tolerance of often negative responses so that the patient experiences no criticism or judgment, then reintegration is seldom possible. Schade agrees with Father Bill in saying that a minister is a companion walking along their ways, the one who stands by, a friend, and leads to an experience of God through prayer, administering the sacraments and scripture, as scriptural affirmations of God constitute the prime source of hope for mentally ill people, and "the Sacraments are visible, tangible expressions of deep religious faith." He adds that to someone who feels rejected by members of his family and by friends and one could add, by parishioners, "the words of the institution of the Supper may convey God's personal interest and concern for the individual" (Schade, 1953: 171, 173).

Murdoch (1994) suggests that the sacrament of Holy Communion appears to be one of the most powerful memory cues and may reassure and calm the most disturbed dementia sufferer. He also advocates that the needs of carers of dementia sufferers must also be remembered by churches and their members, and that their spiritual, physical, emotional, recreational and respite needs must be recognized and addressed within wider church families.

I finally took my mother to see Father Joseph confidentially, on his invitation, when the family thought she was visiting me.

Mom and I spent two hours sitting in Father Joseph's front room while he listened patiently to her outpourings, with some prompting from me. At times I held her hand, as she was very nervous. It was painful for me. She was severely tortured with this well-hidden illness. I knew in my own way I was almost as broken as she and Elizabeth. I had soaked up so much of their suffering.

Father Joseph ministered the sacrament of the sick to us both. I was deeply moved. At last my need was being recognized. No one knows the suffering of people with these hidden illnesses. I had spent years listening to my mother's cries for help, and had carried my daughter through her illness this last year feeling more and more alone, while most others seemed oblivious. Carers, I felt, were the unseen partners (Hunneysett, 2009).

A lady, who attended our pastoral support group for a short while, gave her thoughts on the role of carer when the wife is seriously ill with depression.

A man having to live with a wife with depression finds life very, very difficult, if not to say almost impossible. The woman he married is now very dependent on him, almost childlike in her behavior. Her personality totally changes at that time. His home, which used to be his sanctuary, is now a place of misery. No longer is the life he now lives with his wife the same as before, in fact almost the opposite. His wife is now totally inconsolable, and he finds it impossible to help her out of the kind of hell she is going through. He can hear her crying and repeating worries over and over and there is nothing he can do about it. This is all very upsetting for him to see his wife in such a distressed state, and no matter how many times he tries to console her he cannot make any difference to her behavior. He may very easily slip into depression himself and what will happen then? There has never been a more important time for the Church to support them than now. When people are physically ill, everyone gives them their support, and rightly so. Not so with mental illness though as people feel too embarrassed to tell anyone because of the terrible stigma attached to it. If only people could see this. Understanding is so very important at this time as families of the persons who have depression need lots of support, more than ever before. Unfortunately there are I think a lot of people who think you should be able to pull yourself out of it. As if you have some choice in the matter; I only wish that were the case. It is like something has locked up your mind and you are no longer responsible for your feelings. All of them are sad, not one happy one left. Jean

Address states that our attitude and what we do to the ill individuals and their families is all important to their wellbeing. Acceptance is the key, acceptance to have compassion for the person with the illness, having the courage no longer to feel shame, to reach out with a telephone call to an ill parishioner, to starting a support group for mentally ill persons or their families, to opening the congregation to a community-wide conference on mental health, and that "as professionals, we must strive to create awareness as the first step" (Address, 2003: 88).

Koenig (2005) says that religious communities can be important sources of support and care for those with serious mental illness, and it is simple kinds of activities that can sometimes make a dramatic difference. He cites pastoring as religious counseling and support, to include possible hospital visits, birthday cards, prayer with the pastor or pastoral staff, discussions about faith, Bible study, or involvement in church-related activities. Maves (1953) agrees with this. He says that to address effectively ministry to mentally ill people, takes the united efforts of clergy and congregation together, and with the local churches acting cooperatively.

Pattison concludes that mentally ill people are a major and central challenge to the churches; they are always with us and their challenge to the churches has been perpetual. He suggests that it could be argued that if the churches fail to express practical compassion to the suffering individuals and their families where there is mental illness, or to make the values of the Kingdom of God a reality in society, then "they are failing in their vocation to carry forward the mission and Gospel of Christ" (Pattison, 1986: 37).

The personal testimonies express all that has been revealed in my survey, and in previous literature and research reported in earlier chapters, and lead me to make the following recommendations.

Recommendations
- Raising awareness and education, especially in Christian congregations both for lay people, ministers and leaders, is fundamental to combat resistance, to change negative perceptions, and to help remove prejudice and stigma.
- Practical expressions of support and friendship towards people with mental illnesses from members in faith communities need particularly to be encouraged.
- The Church needs to consider improving benefits by reducing undue demands on or criticism of vulnerable church members.
- The churches' religious programmes need to be complemented by mental health promotional material and by weekend seminars and educational workshops; and the churches' privileged position of ministry could be extended to certain mental health concerns facing members of congregations.
- Needs of carers should be addressed with maximum religious and spiritual support.

- Religious resources should be better understood and more widely used by people with mental ill health, as mental health care can be truly holistic when religious, spiritual and cultural needs of people are taken into account.
- Churches should be mental health promoters particularly in the continuous challenge to stigmatisation and discrimination in society.

If these recommendations were implemented, then people with mental illnesses, their families and carers, would be given more support within Christian congregations, both spiritually and practically. This would allow those experiencing the illnesses to be more integrated into their faith communities and ultimately within society in general, and consequently be of benefit to all of society.

I conclude my writing with Nick's contribution. Nick is divorced with two adult sons and is a granddad. He developed bipolar affective disorder around the age of forty-five and had to give up work. Nick has a very positive attitude about his disorder. He was commissioned as a reader in church many years after he was diagnosed with his illness and was told that he is a good reader. He turned his back on this ministry when he found that the passages and the messages that he felt were for him, "spooked him out," but he is aware that it was his illness. When feeling more confident again, he asked to meet up with me to discuss how he might return to being a reader, as his five-year commissioning had ended.

When at a low ebb, he shuts himself away from the world, but stays within his home sanctuary where he can pray. He told me that he has never been afraid to show

Pastoral Care: Mental Health

his face to the public. He said that his mental illness can happen to any one and there is nothing to be ashamed of, and with good insight into it, it can be self-managed. He wrote a poem that I think speaks of his positive attitude.

Your strength Lord, is within us

When the pressures of life are just too much
We just can't cope and really loose touch
From our illness there is no immunity
But you know we need your community
The people out there are our sisters and brothers
And what has happened to us will happen to others
This is your strength within us, Lord. We know it
We have your gift of compassion to show it
We pray to you, that we use it to benefit others
Your Church and our sisters and brothers
Positive attitude to mental health awareness
Why the stigma? Where's the fairness?
Lord, we believe we understand the position
Give us your strength to work on this mission
AMDG
(Ad Majorem Dei Gloriam: To the greater glory of God)
Nick

Bibliography

Achtemeier PJ gen ed (1985) *Harper's Bible Dictionary*. Harper and Row, San Francisco

Address RF (2003) *Caring for the Soul R'fuat HaNfesh: A Mental Health Resource and Study Guide*. UAHC Press, New York

Alisky JM, Iczkowski K (1990) Barriers to housing for deinstitutionalized psychiatric patients. *Hosp Comm Psychiatry* **41**: 93-95

Allderidge P (1985) Bedlam: fact or fantasy. In: Bynum WF, Porter R, Shepherd M eds. *The Anatomy of Madness Vol. II: Institutions and Society*. Tavistock Publications, London: 17-33

American Association of Pastoral Counselors Pastoral Counseling: A National Mental Health Resource. http://aapc.org/nmhr (13 January 2004)

American Psychiatric Association (1994) *DSM-IV Diagnostic and Statistical Manual of Mental Disorders*, 4th edn. American Psychiatric Association, Washington

Amici Curiae Christian Legal Society and Christian Medical Association (2002) United States Court of Appeals for the Ninth Circuit. http://www.clsnet.org/clrfPages/amicus/ashcroft.pdf (13 January 2004)

Aquinas T (1975) *Summa Theologiae, 57, Baptism and Confirmation*. Blackfriars, London

Aquinas T (1969) *Summa Theologiae, 25, Sin*. Blackfriars, London

Aquinas T (1964) Summa Theologiae, 13, Man Made to God's Image. Blackfriars, London

Association For Pastoral Care In Mental Health Association For Pastoral Care In Mental Health. http://www.pastoral.org.uk/ (30 July 2004)

Association For Pastoral Care In Mental Health (1996) *With a little help from my Friends... Working together for Mental Health*. The Bishop's House, Ely

Association of Christian Counselors Association of Christian Counselors. http://website.lineone/-accord/ACC-Home-Page.htm (18 February 2004)

Avalos H (1999) *Health Care and the Rise of Christianity*. Hendrikson Publishers, Massachusetts

Avalos H (1995) *Illness and Health Care in the Ancient Near East*. The President and Fellows of Harvard College, Scholars Press, Georgia

Batty D (2001) Exorcism: abuse or care. http://s_Hlt4677482861_Hlt487742862oBM_1_BM_2_ciety.guardian.co.uk/mentalhealth/story/0,8150,536719,00.htmi (11 September 2002)

Barham P (1992) *Closing the Asylum: The Mental Patient in Modern Society*. Penguin Books, London

Bennett O (1997) Spirituality: a Christian path. *Nursing Times* **93**(40): 38

Bettinson H (1972) *St Augustine: The City of God* (a new trans). Penquin Books, London

Bishop John Robinson Fellowship (undated) Bishop John Robinson Fellowship, London

Blazdell J (1999) User-led Research in Mental Health. Updates 1 (8) http://www.mentalhealth.org.uk/html/content/update8.cfm (16 February 2003)

Booth G (1953) Health from the Standpoint of the Physician. In: Maves PB ed. *The Church and Mental Health*. Charles Scribner's Sons, New York. London: 3-17

Borinstein AB (1992) Public attitudes towards people with mental illness. *Health Affairs* Fall: 186-196

Boutwood J (2002) Celebrating The Voices Around Us. Association For Pastoral Care In Mental Health Newsletter October http//:www.iop.kcl.ac/main/default.htm (16 February 2003)

Bowling A 1997) *Research Methods in Health*. Open University Press, Buckingham

Bruder EE (1953) In The Mental Hospital. In: Maves PB ed. *The Church and Mental Health*. Charles Scribner's Sons, New York. London: 175-189

Building Partnerships (2001) Black majority churches and mental health services. Building partnerships: mental health services and the faith communities 1 http://www.kingsfund.org.uk/pdf/BuildingPartnerships.pdf (17 January 2004)

Bynum WF, Porter R, Shepherd M eds (1988) The Anatomy of Madness Vol. III: The Asylum and its Psychiatry. Routledge, London

Bynum WF, Porter R, Shepherd M eds (1985) *The Anatomy of Madness Vol. II: Institutions and Society*. Tavistock Publications, London

Byrne P (2001) Psychiatric stigma. In: Crown S, Lee A eds. Reading about. *Br J Psychiatry* **178:** 281-284

Byrne P (2000) Stigma of mental illness and ways of diminishing it. *Adv Psychiatr Treat* **6**: 65-72

Carers Christian Fellowship Carers Christian Fellowship. http://www.carerschristianfellowship.org.uk/index.html (30 July 2004)

Chaplin R (2000) Psychiatrists can cause stigma too. In: Hotopf M ed. Correspondence. *Br J Psychiatry* **177**: 467

Christian C ed (1991) In the Spirit of Truth: A reader in the work of Frank Lake. Darton, Longman and Todd, London

Church of England Guilford Diocese Section 1: Attitudes "*Friends, you must never disparage one another*" James 3, verse 11. http://wwwcofeguilford.org.uk/social-responsibility/opentoall/OpenToAll-Attitudes.pdf (13 January 2004)

Clay RM (1909) *The Medieval Hospitals of England*. Methuen, London

Community-Care carers@communitycare.org.uk Making Space. http://dialspace.dial.pipex.com/prod/dialspace/town/way/glc04/making-space/ (3 March 2004)

Copsey N (2002) *Spiritual And Cultural Care in East London*. http://www.rcpsych.ac.uk/college/sig/spirit/publication/index.htm (17 February 2003)

Corrigan PW *et al* (2001) Prejudice, social distance, and familiarity with mental illness. *Schizophrenia Bull* **27**(2): 219-225

Crisp AH (1999) The stigmatization of sufferers with mental disorders. *Br J Gen Pract* **49**: 3-4

Crisp AH *et al* (2000) Stigmatization of people with mental illnesses. *Br J Psychiatry* **177**: 4-7 http://intl-bjp.rcpsych.org/cgi/content/full/177/1/4 (31 October 2001)

Cule J (1997) The History of Medicine. In: Porter R consultant ed. *Medicine: A History of Healing Ancient Traditions to Modern Practices*. Marlowe and Company, New York: 12-41

Davis J A (2000) *Pastoral care of the Mentally Ill: A Handbook for Pastors*. Universal Publishers/uPUBLISH.com. USA

Department of Health Attitudes to Mental Illness Summary Report 2000. http://www.doh.uk/public/mentalillness.htm (13 August 2003a)

Department of Health National statistics on adults' attitudes to mental illness in Great Britain 2003. http://www.info.doh.gov.uk/doh/intpress.nsf/page/2003-0239?OpenDocument (13 August 2003b)

Department of Health (2000) *Attitudes to Mental Illness Survey: Fieldwork 1-5 March 2000: Tabulations*. Taylor Nelson Sofres RSGB, London

Department of Health (1997) *Attitudes to Mental Illness Summary Report 1997*. RSGB Omnibus, TNS House, London

Digby A (1985) Moral Treatment at the Retreat 1796-1846. In: Bynum WF, Porter R, Shepherd M eds. *The Anatomy of Madness Vol. II: Institutions and Society*. Tavistock Publications, London: 52-72

Dominguez EJ (1967) The Hospital of Innocents: humane treatment of the mentally ill in Spain, 1409-1512. *Bulletin-Menninger Clinic* **31**: 285-297

Dring M (2000) Spirituality in mental health care and nurse training. *Bishop John Robinson Fellowship Newsletter* **18**: 4-7

Dunn S (1999) *Creating Accepting Communities*. Mind Publications, London

Editors (1999) *The Chambers Dictionary*, new edn. Softback Preview. Chambers Harrap Publishers Ltd, Edinburgh

Edwards A, Talbot R (1994) The Hard-Pressed Researcher: A Research Book for the Caring Professions. Longman Group, Essex

Ellison CG, Levin JS (1998) The religion-health connection: evidence, theory, and future directions. *Health Educ Behav* **25**(6): 700-720

Emdon T (1997) Spirituality: cry freedom. *Nurs Times* **93**(40): 35-38

Faulkner A (2000) Strategies for Living. Updates **2**(3) http://www.mentalhealth.org.uk/html/content/updatev02i03.cfm (16 February 2003)

Faulkner A, Layzell S (2000) Strategies for Living: The Research Report. http://www.mentalhealth.org.uk/html/content/s41reportsum.cfm (16 February 2003)

Flannery A gen ed (1987) *Vatican Council II: The Conciliar and Post Conciliar Documents,* study edn. Costello, New York

Flannery A gen ed (1982) *Vatican Council II: More Post Conciliar Documents,* new rev edn. Costello, New York

Foskett J (2000) Souls searching. *Bishop John Robinson Fellowship Newsletter* November/December: 18-19

Friedli L (2000) A matter of faith, religion and mental health. *Int J Ment Health Prom* **2**(2): 7-13

Gill R (1999) *Churchgoing and Christian Ethics*. Cambridge University Press, Cambridge

Goffman E (1963) *Stigma: Notes On The Management Of Spoiled Identity*. Prentice-Hall Inc, New Jersey

Goffman E (1968) *Stigma: Notes On The Management Of Spoiled Identity.* Penquin Books Ltd, London

Graham TF (1967) *Medieval Minds: Mental Health in the Middle Ages*. George Allen and Unwin, London

Gray A (2001) Attitudes of the public to mental health: a church congregation. *Ment Health Relig Cult* **4**(1): 71-79

Grove B (2002) Editorial. *A life in the day* **6**(3): 4

Haghighat R (2001) A unitary theory of stigmatization: pursuit of self-interest and routes to destigmatization. *Br J Psychiatry* **178**: 207-215

Hall J (1997) Spirituality: the search inside. *Nurs Times* **93**(40): 36-37

Hammaker RG (1998) Church: an overlooked mental health resource. *J Relig Health* **37**(1 Spring): 37-44

Hayward P, Bright JA (1997) Stigma and mental illness: a review and critique. *J Mental Health* **6**(4): 345-354

Head J (2002) From the editor. *Bishop John Robinson Fellowship* **13**: 1

Health Education Authority (1999) *Promoting Mental Health: The Role of Faith Communities-Jewish and Christian Perspectives*. Health Education Authority, London

Health Matters (99/00) All the lonely people. Health Matters **39**: Winter http://www.healthmatters.org.uk/stories/dunn.html (26 April 2003)

Hiltner S (1953) Developing a More Effective Chaplaincy Service. In: Maves PB ed. *The Church and Mental Health*. Charles Scribner's Sons, New York. London: 231-238

Holmes M ed (2002) *Way of Life* **34**(1): 1-36

Howe RL (1953) A More Adequate Training for Ministers. In: Maves PB ed. *The Church and Mental Health*. Charles Scribner's Sons, New York. London: 239-252

Hunneysett E (2009) *Our Suicidal Teenagers: Where are you God?* Chipmunkapublishing, London

Hunneysett E (1998) Support for Carers especially of People with Mental Illness and Church Involvement. MA dissertation: Maryvale Institute, Birmingham unpublished

Hunneysett E (1994) The voice of a carer. *Priests and People* **8**(3): 118

Hunter R, MacAlpine I (1963) *Three Hundred Years of Psychiatry 1535-1860*. Oxford University Press, London

Pastoral Care: Mental Health

Jackson SW (1972) Unusual mental states in medieval Europe. *J History Med Allied Sci* **27**: 262-297

John Paul II (2001) Plea for the mentally ill. *The Universe*. 15 April: 11

John Paul II (1994) *Catechism of the Catholic Church*. Geoffrey Chapman, London

Jones K (1993) *Asylums and After: A Revised History of the Mental Health Services: From the Early 18th Century to the 1990s*. The Athlone Press, London

Kaminski P, Harty C (1999) From stigma to strategy. *Nurs Stand* **13**(38): 36-40

Kleinman A (1988) The Illness Narratives: Suffering, Healing and The Human Condition. Basic Books, New York

Kleinman A (1980) Patients and Healers in the Context of Culture: An Exploration of the Borderland between Anthropology, Medicine and Psychiatry. University of California Press, London

Koenig, Harold G (2005) *Faith and Mental Health: Religious Resources for Healing*. Templeton Foundation Press, Philadelphia and London

Koenig HG snr ed (1997) *Is Religion Good for Your health? The Effects of Religion on Physical and Mental Health*. The Haworth Pastoral Press, New York. London

Larson EJ, Amundsen DW (1998) *A Different Death: Euthanasia and the Christian Tradition*. Intervarsity Press, Illinois

Lerner P (1997) Healing and the Mind. In: Porter R consultant ed. *Medicine A History of Healing Ancient Traditions to Modern Practices*. Marlowe and Company, New York: 144-167

Link BG *et al* (1999) Public conceptions of mental illness: labels, causes, dangerousness, and social distance. *Am J Pub Health* **89**(9): 1328-33

Lipsedge M (1996) Religion and madness in history. In: Bhugra D ed. *Psychiatry and Religion: Context, Consensus and Controversies*. Routledge, London: 23-47

Littlewood R, Lipsedge M (1995) Ethnic minorities and the psychiatrist. In: Davey B, Gray A, Seale C eds. *Health and Disease: A Reader,* 2nd edn. Open University Press, Buckingham: 50-54

Livingstone EA ed (1990) *The Concise Oxford Dictionary of the Christian Church,* 2nd edn. abridged. University Press, Oxford

Lowther J (1999) Mental Health: Cinderella in the Developing World. *MMA HealthServe Mobilising Christian Health Care Mission* **7.** http://www.healthserve.org/print/p0015.htm (17 January 2004)

MacDonald M (1981) *Mystical Bedlam: Madness, Anxiety and Healing in Seventeenth Century England.* Cambridge University Press, Cambridge

Marriage and Family Life Project Office of the Catholic Bishops' Conference of England and Wales (2006) What is life like if you or someone in your family has a mental health problem... and what can your family do to make a difference? Catholic Bishops' Conference of England and Wales, London

Marx R ed (1995) Breakthrough. *Breakthrough* **1**: 2

Maves PB ed (1953) *The Church and Mental Health.* Charles Scribner's Sons, New York. London

McKay D (2000) Stigmatizing pharmaceutical advertisements. In: Hotopf M ed. Correspondence. *Br J Psychiatry* **177**: 467-468

McKie A, Swinton J (2000) Community, culture and character: the place of the virtues in psychiatric nursing practice. *J Psychiatr Mental Health Nurs* **7**: 35-42

McNeill JT (1953) Religious Healing of Soul and Body: An Historical Survey. In: Maves PB ed. *The Church and Mental Health.* Charles Scribner's Sons, New York. London: 43-60

McSherry W (2000) Making sense of Spirituality in Nursing Practice: an interactive approach. Churchill Livingstone, London

Mental Health Foundation Mental Health Foundation. http://www.mentalhealth.org.uk/page.cfm?pagecode=OWTF (8 August 2004)

Mental Health Matters (1997) *Families and Friends* Spring: 1-4

Mentality (2001) Making It Happen: A Guide to delivering Mental Health Promotion Department of Health Publications, London

Mentality Mentality: promoting mental health. http://www.mentality.org.uk/about/what.htm (27 July 2004)

Mind (1991) *Understanding Mental Handicap.* Mind Publications, London

Murdoch P (1994) Spiritual needs of dementia sufferers. *Wellsprings* December

Neugebauer R (1978) Treatment of the mentally ill in medieval and early modern England: a reappraisal. *J Hist Behavl Sci* **14**: 158-169

Newcastle Diocesan Board for Mission and Social Responsibility (1996) *I am not an Illness.* Newcastle Diocesan Board for Mission and Social Responsibility, Newcastle

Nicholls V (2002a) Spirituality and Mental Health. Updates **4**(6) Mental Health Foundation, London

Nicholls V ed (2002b) *Taken Seriously: The Somerset Spirituality Project.* Mental Health Foundation, London

Nicholls V (2001) Real Life Evidence in Mental Health. http://www.mentalhealth.org.uk/htm/content/articlemh 15.cfm (16 January 2003)

Nolan P, Crawford P (1997) Towards a rhetoric of spirituality in mental health care. *J Adv Nurs* **26**: 289-294

Nooney J, Woodrum E (2002) Religious coping and church-based social support as predictors of mental health outcomes: testing a conceptual model. *J Scientif Stud Relig* **41** (2): 359-368

Nuffield Council on Bioethics Nuffield Council on Bioethics. http://www.nuffieldbioethics.org/home/index.asp (8 April 2003)

Nuffield Council on Bioethics (1998) *Mental Disorders and Genetics: The Ethical Context*. Nuffield Council on Bioethics, London. http://www.nuffieldbioethics.org/home/index.asp (8 April 2003)

O'Grady TJ (1996) Attitudes to mental illness. *Br J Psychiatry* **168**: 652

ONS Omnibus (1998) ONS Omnibus Survey M 208 Mental Illness and Stigma. On Your Doorstep: Community organisations and mental health. www.scmh.org.uk (4 February 2002)

Oxley GW (1974) *Poor Relief in England and Wales 1601-1834*. David and Charles, London

Papadopoulos C, Leavey G, Vincent C (2002) Factors influencing stigma: a comparison of Greek-Cypriot and English attitudes towards mental illness in north London. *Soc Psychiatry* **37**: 430-434

Pathways to Promise Ministry and Mental Health (1999). http://www.pathwaystopromise.org/resporces/index.htm (3 March 2007)

Pattison S (1993) *A Critique of Pastoral Care,* 2nd edn. SCM Press, London

Pattison S (1989) *Alive and Kicking: Towards a Practical Theology of Illness and Healing*. SCM Press, London

Pattison S (1986) Mentally ill people: a challenge to the churches. *Modern Churchman* **68**: 28-38

Paykel S, Hart D, Priest RG (1998) Changes in public attitudes to depression during the Defeat Depression Campaign. *Br J Psychiatry* **173**: 519-522

Philo G (1994) Media images and popular beliefs. *Psychiatr Bull* **18**: 173-174

Porter R (1998) Can the stigma of mental illness be changed? *Lancet* **352**: 1049-1050

Porter R (1997) The Greatest Benefit to Mankind: A Medical History of Humanity from Antiquity to the Present. Harper Collins Publishers, London

Porter R (1987) *A Social History of Madness*. Weiden and Nicholson, London

Pozner A (2002) Working it out. *A Life in the Day* **6**(3): 4

Puffer KA, Miller KJ (2001) The church as an agent of help in the battle against late life depression. *Pastoral Psychol* **50**(2 November): 125-136

Qvarsell R (1985) Locked up or put to bed: psychiatry and the treatment of the mentally ill in Sweden 1800-1920. In: Bynum WF, Porter R, Shepherd M eds. *The Anatomy of Madness Vol. II: Institutions and Society*. Tavistock Publications, London: 86-97

Rahner K, Vorgrimler H (1983) *The Concise Theological Dictionary,* 2nd edn. Burns and Oates, London

Reda S (1995) Attitudes towards community mental health care of residents in North London. *Psychiatr Bull* **19**: 731-733

Retreat Association (2002) Retreats 2002: Programme and Events for over 200 Retreat Centers. Retreat Association, Newbury

Richardson A, Bowden J eds (1983) *A New Dictionary of Christian Theology*. SCM, London

Richardson CC (1953) The Formal Rites and Ceremonies of the Church. In: Maves PB ed. *The Church and Mental Health*. Charles Scribner's Sons, New York. London: 97-107

Rogers EM (1996) The field of health communication today: an up-to-date report. *J Health Comm Today* **1**: 15-23

Rolheiser R (2003) Is suicide a sin or really a sickness? *Catholic Herald* 10 August: 14

Rose D (1996) *Living in the Community*. Sainsbury Center for Mental Health, London

Sainsbury Center for Mental Health (2001) Forward in Faith. The Guardian 21 February. http://www.scmh.org.uk/802569840056E832/vWeb/wpASTN4_Hlt78794418UBM_13_MEM?_HLT78794368oBM_14_pendocument (17 February 2003a)

Sainsbury Center for Mental Health Sainsbury Center for Mental Health. http://www.scmh.org.uk/802569840056E832/vwA11DocsNews?Open_Hlt78794362VBM_15_iew (16 November 2003b)

SANE About SANE. http://www.sane.org.uk/About-SANE/About.htm (3 March 2004)

SANE (1996) *Sanetalk*. Summer: 1-16

Schade HC (1953) In the Parish. In: Maves PB ed. *The Church and Mental Health*. Charles Scribner's Sons, New York. London: 161-173

Scull A (1993) The Most Solitary of Afflictions: Madness and Society in Britain 1700-1900. Yale University Press, London

Shorter E (1997) *A History of Psychiatry*. John Wiley and Sons, Chichester

Slack P (1988) Poverty and Policy in Tudor and Stuart England. Longman, London

Social Welfare Committee of the Catholic Bishops' Conference of England and Wales (2000) *Dementia – who cares?* Catholic Bishops' Conference of England and Wales, London

Southwark Diocese Board For Social Responsibility Mental Health Working Group (1992) *Travelling Together.... Towards Mental Health*. Southwark Diocese Board For Social Responsibility, Southwark

Sussman S (1997) The community's response to mentally ill people. *Br Med J* **314**: 458

Sutherland M (1999) Towards dialogue: an exploration of the relations between psychiatry and religion in contemporary mental health. In: Woodward J *et al* eds. *The Blackwell Reader in Pastoral Theology*. Blackwell Press, Oxford: 272-282

Swinton J (2001a) Building a church for strangers. *J Relig, Disabil Health* **4**(4): 25-63

Swinton J (2001b) Spirituality and Mental Health Care: Rediscovering a "Forgotten" Dimension. Jessica Kinglsey Publishers, London

Swinton J (2000) Resurrecting the Person: Friendship and the Care of People With Mental Health Problems. Abingdon Press, Nashville

Swinton J (1997a) From Bedlam to Shalom: Towards a Practical Theology of Human Nature, Interpersonal Relationships and Mental Health Care. PhD thesis: University of Aberdeen, Aberdeen: 30-31 unpublished

Swinton J (1997b) Restoring the image: spirituality, faith, and cognitive disability. *J Relig Health* **36**(1 Spring): 21-27

Swinton J, Kettles AM (1997) Resurrecting the person: redefining mental illness–a spiritual perspective. *Psychiatr Care* **4**(3): 118-121

Tees and North East Yorkshire NHS Trust (2003) Modernisation of Mental Health and Learning Disability Services. *Ad>ance* **5**

Tees and North East Yorkshire NHS Trust (2002) Trust's Campaign to tackle stigma. *Trust Bull* **47**

Tees, Durham and Darlington Health Promotion Consortium (2004) *Certificate in Promoting Mental Well-Being.* North Tees PCT Health Promotion Service, Stockton

Toner PJ (2003) Exorcism. In: Knight K ed. *The Catholic Encyclopedia* (online edition). http://www.newadvent.org/cathen/05709a.htm (20 March 2004)

Truscott F (1995) *Coping with...Mental Illness.* CTS Publications, London

University of Durham Information Technology Service (1999) *SPSS for Windows NT/95/98.* University of Durham Information Technology Service, Durham

Vallat J (1999) The Chairman's Letter. *Association For Pastoral Care In Mental Health Newsletter* July: 1

Vatican City (2005) ZENIT.org

Verne A (1961) *Fugitive Saint.* The Catholic Printing Company, Bolton

Warner R (2001) Community attitudes towards mental disorder. In: Thornicroft G, Szmukler G eds. *Textbook of Community Psychiatry* University Press, Oxford: 453-464

White PD (1998) Changing minds: banishing the stigma of mental illness. *J Roy Soc Med* **91**(10): 509-510

Wilcox C (1998) *Finding out for yourself: DIY surveys.* North of England Institute for Christian Education, Durham

Wilmer HA, Scammon RE (1954) Neuropsychiatric patients reported cured at St. Bartholomew's Hospital in the twelfth century: selected cases from the Book of Foundation of St Bartholomew's Church in London. *J Nervous Mental Dis* **119**(1): 1-22

Wolff G *et al* (1996a) Community attitudes to mental illness. *Br J Psychiatry* **168**: 183-190

Wolff G *et al* (1996b) Community knowledge of mental illness and reaction to mentally ill people. *Br J Psychiatry* **168**: 191-198

Wolff G *et al* (1996c) Public education for community care: a new approach. *Br J Psychiatry* **168**: 441-447

Woodward LE (1953) Fostering Mental Health through the Church Program. In: Maves PB ed. *The Church and Mental Health.* Charles Scribner's Sons, New York. London: 129-157

World Health Organisation (1992) The ICD - 10 Classification of Mental and Behavioural Disorders: Clinical descriptions and diagnostic guidelines. World Health Organisation, Geneva

Wright S (1997) Spirituality: the awakening. *Nurs Times*: **93** (40): 34